Antiepileptic Drugs, Pharmacopoeia

C.P. Panayiotopoulos

Antiepileptic Drugs, Pharmacopoeia

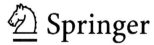 Springer

C.P. Panayiotopoulos MD, PhD, FRCP
Department of Clinical Neurophysiology and Epilepsies
St. Thomas Hospital
London SE1 7EH
United Kingdom
and
Department of Neurosciences
John Radcliffe Hospital
Oxford OX3 9DU
United Kingdom

ISBN 978-0-85729-011-3
Springer London Dordrecht Heidelberg New York

A catalogue record for this book is available from the British Library

Library of Congress Control Number: 2010936356

Cover design: eStudio Calamar S.L.

Printed on acid-free paper

Springer is part of Springer Science+Business Media (www.springer.com)

Contents

Abbreviations

ADR	adverse drug reaction	IGE	idiopathic generalised epilepsy abbreviations
AED	anti-epileptic drug	IL	interleukin
CI	confidence interval	IV	intravenous
CNS	central nervous system	JME	juvenile myoclonic epilepsy
CRMP	collapsin response mediator protein	MCM	major congenital malformation
CSF	cerebrospinal fluid	NMDA	N-methyl d-aspartate
CSWS	continuous spike-and-wave during sleep	PCR	polymerase chain reaction
CTS	centrotemporal spike	PEHO	progressive encephalopathy with edema, hypsarrhythmia and optic atrophy
CYP	cytochrome P450	PI	package insert
ECG	electocardiogram	RCT	randomised controlled trial
EEG	electroencephalogram	SmPC	Summary of Product Characteristics
EMEA	European Medicines Agency	SUDEP	sudden unexpected death in epilepsy
FDA	US Food & Drug Administration	SV2A	synaptic vesicle protein 2A
GABA	Gamma-aminobutyric acid	TDM	therapeutic drug monitoring
GABA-T	GABA-transaminase	UGT	uridine diphosphate glucuronosyltransferase
GTCS	generalised tonic–clonic seizure		
HLA	human leukocyte antigen		

Introduction

This pharmacopoeia is mainly based on information provided by package inserts (PIs) in accordance with US Food and Drug Administration (FDA) approval and the Summary of Product Characteristics (SmPC) of the European Medicines Agency (EMEA) for each drug used in prophylactic treatment of recurrent epileptic seizures. Although this information is supplemented by extensively cited, recently published reports and expert clinical advice, it is not intended as a substitute for the PI or SmPC, which are the legal, most complete sources of information on a drug. Rather, this concise guide provides the properties and clinical applications of each antiepileptic drug (AED) in a user-friendly template that physicians may consult to best treat patients with epileptic seizures. The authorised indications in the SmPC and PI are current as of May 2010.

This is a pharmacopoeia of all AEDs currently used in the prophylactic treatment of epileptic seizures around the world, including older and the newest-generation AEDs. Most of these AEDs have authorised indications in the United States (FDA-PI) and Europe (EMEA-SmPC), which may be different; in fact, some AEDs are licensed in Europe but not in the United States (e.g., clobazam) or vice versa (e.g., felbamate). Further, in Europe, some AEDs, such as valproate, phenytoin, and lamotrigine, do not have a centrally approved license by the European Commission, and each country in which an AED is licensed in Europe may have slightly different licensed indications. In these cases, the information provided is from the UK-SmPC. In addition, some AEDs, such as sulthiame, are licensed in some countries through local regulatory authorities but do not have EMEA or FDA approval.

There is a constant flow of information relating to AED therapy, especially for adverse drug reactions, interactions with other drugs, and warnings and precautions that may impact labelling. Therefore, physicians should consult the authorised indications and product information found in the approved prescribing information for the country in which they practice medicine before making a decision as to whether a particular AED is appropriate for their patients.

Recommended sources of information

For information regarding the PI and SmPC of AEDs, some suggestions have been made. The package insert (PI) can be obtained from http://dailymed.nlm. nih.gov/dailymed/about.cfm. The summary of product characteristics (SmPC) can be obtained in any European language from http://www.emea.europa.eu/ htms/human/epar/a.htm. In the UK these are also available from http://emc. medicines.org.uk.

Information about clinical trials (purpose, who may participate, locations, and phone numbers for more details) may be searched for in http://www.clinicaltrials. gov. ClinicalTrials.gov is a registry of federally and privately supported clinical trials conducted in the United States and around the world.

The Handbook of Epilepsy Treatment[1] by Simon Shorvon is highly recommended. The synonymously titled books, Treatment of Epilepsy,[2,3] and Pediatric Epilepsy: Diagnosis and Treatment[4] are other recommended sources that provide more detailed AED information.

AEDs in development and updates on newer AEDs have been recently detailed by the Ninth Eilat conference held in June, 2008.[5]

Acetazolamide

Acetazolamide, an heterocyclic sulfonamide, is a carbonic anhydrase-inhibiting drug used predominantly for the treatment of glaucoma.

Authorised indications

UK-SmPC: second-line drug for both tonic–clonic and focal seizures. It is occasionally helpful in atypical absence, atonic and tonic seizures.
FDA-PI: adjunctive treatment of centrencephalic epilepsies (petit mal, unlocalised seizures).

Clinical applications

Acetazolamide has limited use as an adjunctive therapy for a variety of seizures, but mainly absences.[6] However, it also controls myoclonic jerks, generalised tonic–clonic seizures (GTCSs) and focal seizures. It is particularly used for intermittent administration in catamenial epilepsy (5 days before the expected onset of menses and continued until termination of bleeding);[7] it is not recommended if there is a likelihood of pregnancy.

Dosage and titration

Adults: start treatment with 250 mg and increase to 500–750 mg.
Children: 10–20 mg/day.
Dosing: two or three times daily.
Therapeutic drug monitoring (TDM): not needed.
Reference range: 10–14 mg/l (400–700 μmol/l).

Main ADRs

Frequent and/or/or important: flushing, lethargy, anorexia, nausea, vomiting, paraesthesiae and increased diuresis.
Serious: idiosyncratic reactions, as with other sulfonamides (rash, aplastic anaemia, Stevens–Johnson syndrome), renal failure; nephrolithiasis in chronic treatment and metabolic acidosis, as with other carbonic anhydrase inhibitors (see also topiramate).

Mechanism of action

Acetazolamide is a carbonic anhydrase-inhibiting drug that reversibly catalyses the hydration of CO_2 and the dehydration of carbonic acid. It blocks the action of brain carbonic anhydrase, resulting in an elevation of intracellular CO_2, a decrease of intracellular pH and depression of neuronal activity.

Pharmacokinetics

Oral bioavailability: >90%.

Protein binding: 90–95%.

Metabolism: does not undergo metabolic alteration.

Excretion: renal.

Elimination half-life: 12–14 hours.

Drug interactions

Not significant: reduces carbamazepine levels; salicylates increase levels of acetazolamide due to competition at the renal tubule for secretion.

Main disadvantages

Unpredictable seizure efficacy, development of tolerance and idiosyncratic reactions that exceptionally may be fatal.

Useful clinical notes

- Risk of withdrawal seizures.
- Combination with carbamazepine or oxcarbazepine increases the risk of hyponatraemia.
- Avoid concurrent use with other carbonic anhydrase inhibitors (i.e. sulthiame, topiramate, zonisamide).
- It should be withdrawn prior to starting a ketogenic diet.
- Concurrent use with aspirin can lead to high plasma concentrations of acetazolamide and toxicity.

Benzodiazepines

2

Benzodiazepines are a group of two-ring heterocyclic compounds consisting of a benzene ring fused to a diazepine ring. The first benzodiazepine, chlordiazepoxide, was introduced in clinical practice as anxiolytic and hypnotic in 1960 under the brand name Librium. Diazepam (Valium) followed in 1963. There are today over 30 benzodiazenines (15 are marketed in the USA) used for anxiety, panic, insomnia, agitation, seizures, muscle spasms, alcohol withdrawal and as a premedication for medical or dental procedures.

In epilepsies:[8,9]

- clobazam (see chapter 4) and clonazepam (see chapter 5) are the most useful of all benzodiazepines for preventing recurrent seizures; clonazepam is the main drug used for myoclonic jerks, whereas clobazam is more effective in focal seizures.
- Nitrazepam is another long-acting benzodiazepine which has been used as an AED, mainly in epileptic encephalopathies and particularly in West syndrome. Its usefulness is very limited because of severe sedative ADRs, sialorroeia, hypotonia, development of tolerance and its low efficacy in relation to other more appropriate AEDs. Nitrazepam is not discussed further in this booklet.
- diazepam, lorazepam and midazolam are exclusively used in the treatment of status epilepticus.

Main ADRs

Sedation (sometimes intolerably severe), drowsiness, fatigue, hypersalivation, behavioural and cognitive impairment, restlessness, aggressiveness and coordination disturbances.

Tolerance, dependence and withdrawal syndrome

Benzodiazepines are addictive and regulated in schedule IV of the US Controlled Substance Act. Long term use is associated with benzodiazepine tolerance, dependence and withdrawal syndrome. Benzodiazepine tolerance manifests with decreasing efficacy over time so that larger doses are required to achieve the same effect as with the original dose. In benzodiazepine dependence a person becomes dependent on benzodiazepines physically, psychologically or both. Benzodiazepine withdrawal is similar to the barbiturate or alcohol withdrawal syndrome. Administration of therapeutic doses of benzodiazepines for 6 weeks or longer can result in physical dependence, characterised by a

C.P. Panayiotopoulos, *Antiepileptic Drugs, Pharmacopoeia*,
© Springer-Verlag London Limited 2011

withdrawal syndrome when the drug is discontinued. With larger doses, the physical dependence develops more rapidly.

Main mechanism of action

GABA$_A$-receptor agonists (see note below).

Useful note

GABAergic AEDs

GABA is the main inhibitory neurotransmitter in the brain. It is synthesised in the presynaptic terminals of inhibitory neurones and degraded by GABA transaminase (GABA-T). Of the GABA receptors, GABA$_A$ and GABA$_C$ are ligand-gated ion channels, whereas GABA$_B$ receptors are G-protein-coupled receptors.

The action of GABAergic AEDs is mainly through the GABA$_A$ (inhibition of most types of epileptic seizure) and GABA$_B$ (activation of absence seizures) receptors.

When GABA binds to GABA$_A$ receptors, chloride (Cl$^-$) channels open and allow increased entry to Cl$^-$ ions, which ultimately cause hyperpolarisation of the neurone or inhibition. There are three basic binding sites to this complex GABA$_A$ receptor; the GABA site, the benzodiazepine site and a barbiturate site within the ion channel. Most drugs affecting the GABA$_A$ receptor act to modulate it rather than to directly excite or inhibit it. This modulation generally acts to increase the probability of the channel opening for a given concentration of GABA, or to increase the time that the receptor remains open. GABA$_A$ receptors are the main binding sites for benzodiazepines and barbiturates. Benzodiazepine derivatives (e.g. clobazam, clonazepam and diazepam) increase the frequency of the Cl$^-$ channel openings, whereas barbiturates (e.g. phenobarbital) prolong the opening time of the Cl$^-$ channel. Both the benzodiazepines and barbiturates also enhance the affinity of the GABA$_A$ receptors for GABA.

The GABA$_B$ receptors are metabotrophic transmembrane receptors for GABA that are linked via G-proteins to potassium channels. Thalamic GABA$_B$ receptors modulate absence seizures. Baclofen, a GABA$_B$ receptor agonist, promotes absence seizures.

Tiagabine and vigabatrin increase GABA and cause non-specific activation of the GABA$_A$ (thus inhibiting seizures) and GABA$_B$ (thus aggravating absences) receptors. The anti-epileptic effect of most other AEDs with GABA-ergic activity (e.g. gabapentin, pregabalin and valproate) is probably in combination with other anti-epileptic properties.

Carbamazepine

3

Carbamazepine is an iminodibenzyl derivative designated chemically as 5H-dibenzo[b,f]azepine 5-carboxamide. It is structurally related to the tricyclic antidepressants. It was first introduced into clinical practice in 1962, mainly for the treatment of trigeminal neuralgia prior to becoming the main AED for focal epilepsies.

Authorised indications

UK-SmPC: Epilepsy – generalised tonic–clonic and partial seizures. Carbamazepine Retard is indicated in newly diagnosed patients with epilepsy and in those patients who are uncontrolled or unable to tolerate their current anti-convulsant therapy.

Note: Carbamazepine is not usually effective in absences (petit mal) and myoclonic seizures. Moreover, anecdotal evidence suggests that seizure exacerbation may occur in patients with atypical absences.

FDA-PI: Carbamazepine is indicated for use as an anticonvulsant drug. Evidence supporting efficacy of carbamazepine as an anticonvulsant was derived from active drug-controlled studies that enrolled patients with the following seizure types:

1 Partial seizures with complex symptomatology (psychomotor, temporal lobe). Patients with these seizures appear to show greater improvement than those with other types.
2 Generalised tonic–clonic seizures (grand mal).
3 Mixed seizure patterns which include the above, or other partial or generalised seizures. Absence seizures (petit mal) do not appear to be controlled by carbamazepine.

Clinical applications

Carbamazepine is the superior drug for the treatment of focal epilepsies of any type (idiopathic or symptomatic) with or without secondarily GTCS. It is also licensed for the treatment of primarily GTCSs. In numerous comparative studies, no other drug showed better efficacy than carbamazepine in focal seizures. However, carbamazepine is ineffective and contraindicated in idiopathic generalised epilepsies (IGEs) and epileptic encephalopathies. It is probably ineffective in neonatal and febrile seizures.

Dosage and titration

'Start low and go slow' is important when initiating carbamazepine treatment in order to minimise ADRs.

Adults and children over 12 years of age: start treatment with 200 mg/day in two equally divided doses and increase at weekly intervals in increments of 200 mg/day up to a total of 800–1200 mg/day. Rarely, higher doses of up to 1800 mg/day are needed.

Children 6–12 years old: start with 100 mg/day in two equally divided doses and increase at weekly intervals in increments of 100 mg/day up to a total of 600–1000 mg/day.

Children under 6 years: start with 10–20 mg/kg/day in two or three divided doses and increase at weekly intervals in increments of 10–20 mg/kg/day up to a maintenance dose of no more than 35 mg/kg/day.

There is a significant difference between the carba-mazepine dose given as monotherapy and that used in combination with other AEDs. Higher doses may be necessary in polytherapy with enzyme-inducing AEDs, which increase the metabolism of carbamazepine.

Dosing: two or three times daily.

Fluctuations in the levels of carbamazepine can be reduced by the use of sustained-release preparations.

The clearance of carbamazepine in children is faster than in adults and therefore three- and, sometimes, four-times daily dosing may be required.

TDM: useful but substantial diurnal variation in plasma concentrations is common and symptoms of toxicity due to carbamazepine epoxide may occur without increases in carbamazepine levels.

Reference range: 3–12 mg/l (12–50 µmol/l). Carbamazepine epoxide: up to 9 µmol/l.

> *Developing diplopia may be a good indicator of maximum tolerated carbamazepine levels or epoxide toxicity when carbamazepine levels are within the target range.*

Main ADRs

Frequent and/or important: sedation, headache, diplopia, blurred vision, rash, gastrointestinal disturbances, ataxia, tremor, impotence, hyponatraemia and neutropenia. CNS-related ADRs are usually dose related and appear on initiation of treatment.

Dose-related reduction in neutrophil count occurs in 10–20% of patients treated with carbamazepine, but it rarely drops below 1.2×10^9. The vast majority of cases of leucopenia have not progressed to the more serious conditions of aplastic anaemia or agranulocytosis. Nonetheless, complete pretreatment haematological testing should be obtained as a baseline. If a patient in the course of treatment exhibits low or decreased white blood cell or platelet counts, the patient should be monitored closely. Discontinuation of the drug should be considered if any evidence for significant bone marrow depression develops.

Hyponatraemia occurs in around 5% of treated patients (see oxcarbazepine). Most physicians advise obtaining blood counts at baseline and every 6–8 weeks for the first 6 months of carbamazepine treatment.

Other: Carbamazepine has shown mild anticholinergic activity; patients with increased intraocular pressure should therefore be warned and advised regarding possible hazards.

Serious: allergic skin rash is the most common idiosyncratic ADR that occurs in 5–10% of patients (probably reduced by half with slow titration of controlled-release carbamazepine). This is usually mild and develops within the first 2–6 weeks of treatment. Carbamazepine should immediately be withdrawn if a skin rash develops in order to prevent serious and sometimes life-threatening conditions, such as anticonvulsant hypersensitivity syndrome. Hepatotoxicity usually occurs in the setting of a generalised hypersensitivity response.

HLA-B*1502[10-13] in individuals of Han Chinese and Thai origin has been shown to be strongly associated with the risk of developing Stevens-Johnson syndrome when treated with carbamazepine. Whenever possible, these individuals should be screened for this allele before starting treatment with carbamazepine. If these individuals test positive, carbamazepine should not be started unless there is no other therapeutic option. Tested patients who are found to be negative for HLA-B*1502 have a low risk of Stevens-Johnson syndrome, although the reactions may still very rarely occur. It is not definitely known whether all individuals of south east-Asian ancestry are at risk due to lack of data. The allele HLA-B*1502 has been shown not to be associated with Stevens-Johnson syndrome in the Caucasian population.

The risk for aplastic anaemia and agranulocytosis is five- to eight-times greater than in the general population, which is very low.

Cardiac conduction disturbances are rare and mainly occur in susceptible patients (those with pre-existing cardiac abnormalities and the elderly). These are re-assessed[14,15] in view of cardiac conduction abnormalities now highlighted with newer AEDs.

> FDA warning: All patients who are currently taking or starting on carbamazepine for any indication should be monitored for notable changes in behaviour that could indicate the emergence or worsening of suicidal thoughts or behaviour or depression.

Considerations in women

Pregnancy: category D. Contrary to previous studies, recent pregnancy registries are consistent in the finding that risk of teratogenicity with carbamazepine is relatively small.[16] In a recent study the major congenital malformation (MCM) rate for pregnancies exposed only to carbamazepine was 2.2% (1.4–3.4%), which is less than the MCM rate for women with epilepsy who had not taken AEDs during pregnancy (3.5% [1.8–6.8%]; n=239).[17]

Main mechanisms of action

Carbamazepine stabilises hyperexcited nerve membranes, inhibits repetitive neuronal discharges, and reduces synaptic propagation of excitatory impulses.

Its main mechanism of action appears to be the prevention of repetitive firing of sodium-dependent action potentials in depolarised neurons via use- and voltage-dependent blockade of sodium channels.

Whereas reduction of glutamate release and stabilisation of neuronal membranes may account for the antiepileptic effects, the depressant effect on dopamine and noradrenaline turnover could be responsible for the antimanic properties of carbamazepine.

Pharmacokinetics

Oral bioavailability: 75–85%. It is unaffected by food intake. Bioavailability may be reduced by up to 50% when stored in hot humid conditions. The slow release formulation shows about 15% lower bioavailability than standard preparations. After oral administration, absorption is relatively slow and often erratic, reaching peak plasma concentrations within 4–24 hours; 75–85% of orally ingested carbamazepine is absorbed. Absorption and bioavailability vary among different carbamazepine formulations. Slow-release formulations show about 15% lower bioavailability than standard preparations and have a prolonged absorption phase. Syrup formulations reach maximum plasma concentration faster than chewable or plain tablets.

> *There are significant diurnal variations in the plasma concentrations of carbamazepine. This is greater in children than in adults, which can result in intermittent ADRs that demand adjustments to the daily dosing.*

Protein binding: 66–89%.

Metabolism: carbamazepine is extensively metabolised in the liver. The predominant elimination pathway leads to the formation of carbamazepine 10,11-epoxide, which is a stable and pharmacologically active agent with its own anti-epileptic activity and ADRs.

Carbamazepine epoxide makes a greater contribution to the pharmacological effects (both beneficial and toxic) of carbamazepine in children than in adults. This is because children metabolise carbamazepine more rapidly than adults and this results in carbamazepine epoxide concentrations approaching those of carbamazepine.

Carbamazepine is a potent enzyme inducer. It also induces its own metabolism (autoinduction) by simulating the activity of the cytochrome P450 (CYP) subenzyme 3A4. Autoinduction is usually completed within 3–5 weeks. The half-life of carbamazepine decreases considerably from 18–55 hours to 6–18 hours as autoinduction takes place. In practical terms, this means that carbamazepine levels fall significantly (by about 50%) after several weeks of treatment, which may result in seizure recurrence within this period of autoinduction.

Elimination half-life: 5–26 hours. In combination treatment, the elimination half-life of carbamazepine is reduced by enzyme inducers and increased by enzyme inhibitors.

Drug interactions[18-20]

With other AEDs

Carbamazepine metabolism is highly inducible by certain AEDs.

Enzyme-inducing AEDs, such as phenobarbital, phenytoin and primidone, cause significant reductions in plasma concentrations of carbamazepine. Furthermore, AEDs exacerbate and often double the diurnal variation of plasma carbamazepine concentrations, thus increasing the risk of transient ADRs.

Valproate markedly increases carbamazepine epoxide levels (sometimes fourfold) without concurrent changes in carbamazepine plasma concentration.

Co-medication with lamotrigine may cause neurotoxic symptoms of headache, nausea, diplopia and ataxia, probably as the result of a pharmacodynamic interaction and not by increasing carbamazepine epoxide (as originally suggested). Conversely, carmabazepine decreases plasma levels of lamotrigine.

Concomitant use of carbamazepine and levetiracetam has been reported to increase carbamazepine-induced toxicity.

With non-AEDs

Major: carbamazepine increases the metabolism and therefore decreases the efficacy of a wide variety of drugs, such as oral contraceptives, theophylline, oral anticoagulants and beta-blockers.

Macrolide antibiotics, such as erythromycin, inhibit carbamazepine metabolism and have been associated with carbamazepine toxicity. Carbamazepine toxicity is observed shortly after starting erythromycin therapy, is rapidly reversed on withdrawal of the antibiotic, but can be severe if not recognised early.

Combination therapy with monoamine oxidase inhibitors should be avoided, because carbamazepine has structural similarities with tricyclic antidepressants. *Potential:* additive cardiotoxicity with calcium channel blockers and beta-blockers.

Main disadvantages

Idiosyncratic and other ADRs, drug–drug interactions, the need for laboratory testing and relatively narrow spectrum of anti-epileptic efficacy.

Although carbamazepine is the best AED in the treatment of focal seizures and secondarily GTCSs, it offers no benefit in most other epilepsies, where it is either ineffective or seizure exacerbating. It exaggerates myoclonic jerks, absences and atonic seizures.[21-23] Exceptionally, carbamazepine may exaggerate seizures in Panayiotopoulos syndrome and rolandic epilepsy and may induce non-convulsive status and features of serious atypical evolutions.[24]

Clobazam

Clobazam was the first 1,5-benzodiazepine and was designed to have a chemical structure with a different pharmacological profile from that of the 1,4-benzodiazepines.

Authorised indications

UK-SmPC: adjunctive therapy in epilepsy.
FDA-PI: not licensed.

Clinical applications

Clobazam is a very useful AED, both as polytherapy and monotherapy.[25-35] It is neglected in current clinical practice, mainly because it is erroneously considered to (1) induce high dependence/tolerance and (2) be of similar effectiveness regarding seizure type to clonazepam.

The main clinical applications of clobazam are:

- Adjunctive medication in all forms of drug-resistant epilepsy in adults and children. It is particularly effective in focal rather than generalised seizures. Clobazam was found to have equivalent efficacy to carbamazepine and phenytoin monotherapy in childhood epilepsies.[25,34]
- Intermittent administration 5 days prior and during the menses in catamenial epilepsy[35] is the most popular textbook recommendation.

The CYP2C19 genotype had an impact on the metabolism, efficacy and ADRs of clobazam.[35,36]

Dosage and titration

Adults and children over 12 years: start treatment with 5–10 mg/day at night and increase at weekly intervals in increments of 5 mg/day up to a total of 40 mg/day. In my experience 10 mg taken before sleep is often therapeutic in focal seizures. I do not use a dose of more than 20 mg in children.
Children under 12 years: start with 0.1–0.2 mg/kg/day and slowly increase at weekly intervals in increments of 0.1 mg/kg/day up to a total of 0.8 mg/kg/day.
Dosing: once or twice daily; a smaller dose in the day time and a larger dose prior to sleep.
TDM: not useful except when unusual ADRs appear.[36]
Reference range: norclobazam (active metabolite) 60–200 µg/l (200–670 nmol/l).

Main ADRs

As for all benzodiazepines, but much milder than with most. Somnolence may be partly prevented by administering the drug in small doses 1 hour prior to going to sleep. The cognitive and behavioural effects of clobazam appear to be similar to those of standard monotherapy with carbamazepine or phenytoin.[25]

Severe aggressive outbursts, hyperactivity, insomnia and depression with suicidal ideation may occur, particularly in children.

Tolerance may develop, but this aspect has been largely overemphasised, as documented in many studies.[37-39] More than a third of patients do not develop tolerance. When clobazam is effective, most patients continue to benefit for years without drug dependence or unwanted ADRs.

Main mechanism of action

GABA$_A$-receptor agonist (see note on page 6).

Pharmacokinetics

Oral bioavailability: 90%.

Protein binding: 85%.

Metabolism: hepatic oxidation and then conjugation. N-desmethyl clobazam (norclobazam) is its principal and active metabolite.

Elimination half-life: 20 hours, but this is about 50 hours of its principal metabolite, norclobazam.

Drug interactions

Minor and not clinically significant. Potentiates the effect of CNS depressants such as alcohol, barbiturates and neuroleptics.

Main disadvantages

Sedation and development of tolerance (though the latter may have been exaggerated).

Useful clinical notes

Clobazam should be tried as adjunctive medication in all drug-resistant epilepsies at a dose of 10–30 mg nocte (half this dose in children >5 years old). It is more effective in focal than generalised epilepsies and can also be used as monotherapy. Probably only one out of ten patients will have a clinically significant improvement, but this may be very dramatic and render the patient seizure-free.

Unlike clonazepam, clobazam is much less effective in myoclonic jerks and absences.

Avoid overmedication. Small doses 10–20 mg given 1 hour prior to going to sleep may be therapeutic and well tolerated.

Withdrawal should be very slow, occurring over months. Rapid discontinuation may lead to withdrawal symptoms, seizures and status epilepticus.

Clonazepam

Clonazepam is a 1,4-benzodiazepine.

Authorised indications

UK-SmPC: all clinical forms of epileptic disease and seizures in infants, children, and adults, especially absence seizures, including atypical absences; primarily or secondarily generalised tonic–clonic, tonic or clonic seizures; focal seizures; various forms of myoclonic seizures, myoclonus and associated abnormal movements.

FDA-PI: alone or as an adjunct in the treatment of the Lennox–Gastaut syndrome (petit mal variant), akinetic and myoclonic seizures. In patients with absence seizures (petit mal) who have failed to respond to succinimides, clonazepam may be useful. Lower age limit is not specified.

Clinical applications

Clonazepam[8,40] is the most effective AED in the treatment of myoclonic jerks (superior to valproate), and is also effective in absences (although much more inferior to valproate and ethosuximide)[6] and focal seizures (it is much more inferior to carbamazepine and any other appropriate drug for this type of seizures). Opinions about its effectiveness in GTCSs are conflicting and range from beneficial[41] to aggrevation.[42]

> *Clonazepam is the main AED for myoclonic jerks in all forms of idiopathic or symptomatic and progressive epilepsies (monotherapy, but mainly adjunctive therapy).*

Clonazepam monotherapy is probably the first choice in reading epilepsy (better than valproate). It is particularly effective in juvenile myoclonic epilepsy (JME) if myoclonic jerks are not controlled by other drugs. Adding small doses of clonazepam (0.5–2 mg prior to going to sleep) to valproate, levetiracetam or lamotrigine is highly beneficial and may prevent an unnecessary increase of the main concomitant drug. It is widely used in epileptic encephalopathies, but may also be responsible for benzodiazepine-related ADRs (e.g. sialorrhoea and lethargy).

Dosage and titration

'Start low and go slow' is essential, both in adults and children.

Adults: start treatment with 0.25 mg/day at night and increase at weekly intervals in increments of 0.25 mg/day up to a total of 8–10 mg/day. In my experience, 0.5–2 mg of clonazepam taken before sleep is often highly effective in controlling myoclonic jerks either as monotherapy or as adjunctive therapy in resistant cases.

Children: start with 0.01–0.02 mg/kg/day and slowly increase up to 0.1–0.2 mg/kg/day.

Dosing: once or twice daily; a smaller dose in the day time and a larger dose prior to going to sleep.

TDM: not needed.

Reference range: 20–80 µg/l (80–250 nmol/l).

Main ADRs

Frequent and/or important: sedation, drowsiness, hypersalivation, hyperactivity, lack of concentration and incoordination. Sedation is more serious than with clobazam. This may be partly prevented by administering the drug in small doses 1 hour prior to going to sleep.

Serious: withdrawal syndrome after chronic use.

  See also benzodiazepines.

Main mechanism of action

$GABA_A$-receptor agonist (see useful note on page 6).

Pharmacokinetics

Oral bioavailability: >80%.
Protein binding: 85%.
Metabolism: hepatic.
Elimination half-life: 20–80 hours.

Drug interactions

Minor and not clinically significant. Potentiates the effect of CNS depressants such as alcohol, barbiturates and neuroleptics.

Main disadvantages

Sedation and development of tolerance.

Useful clinical notes

- Clonazepam is the first-choice drug for the control of myoclonic jerks (either as monotherapy if this is the only seizure type, as in reading epilepsy, or mainly as adjunctive medication).

- Avoid overmedication. Small doses 1 hour prior to sleep may be effective and well tolerated.

- Withdrawal should be very slow, occuring over months. A rapid discontinuation often leads to withdrawal symptoms, seizures and status epilepticus.

Eslicarbazepine acetate[43–45]

Eslicarbazepine acetate [(S)-(--)-10-acetoxy-10,11-dihydro-5H-dibenz[b,f]azepine-5-carboxamide] is a prodrug of eslicarbazepine (S-9-(-)-10-acetoxy-10,11-dihydro-5H-dibenz/b,f/azepine-5-carboxamide) and shares with carbamazepine and oxcarbazepine the dibenzazepine nucleus bearing the 5-carboxamide substitute, but is structurally different at the 10,11-position. Eslicarbazepine acetate is the latest AED to be licensed in Europe (April 2009) with the brand names Exalief and Zebinix (it will trade in USA as Stedesa).

Authorised indications
SmPC. Adjunctive therapy in adults (≥ 18 years of age) within the treatment of focal seizures with or without secondary generalisation.
FDA. Not yet licensed.

Clinical applications
Eslicarbazepine acetate is the newest AED licensed for adjunctive treatment of focal seizures. Considering its similarities with carbamazepine, eslicarbazepine acetate may be contra-indicated in generalised seizures, though this has not been assessed.

Dosage and titration
Adults. The recommended starting dose is 400 mg once daily which should be increased to 800 mg once daily after one or two weeks. Based on individual response, the dose may be increased to 1200 mg once daily.
Dosing. Once daily.
Therapeutic drug monitoring. Unknown.
Reference range. Unknown.

Main ADRs
Frequent and/or important. Dizziness, somnolence, headache, ataxia, inattention, diplopia, tremor, nausea, vomiting.
Serious. Rash in 1.1% and hyponatraemia in 1% of total treated population.
The use of eslicarbazepine acetate is associated with increase in the PR interval. Adverse reactions associated with PR interval prolongation that include atrioventricular block, syncope and bradycardia may occur. No second or higher degree atrioventricular block was seen.

Considerations in women
Pregnancy. Category C. Studies in animals have shown reproductive toxicity.

Breastfeeding. Unknown but possibly excreted in breast milk (animal data).
Interactions with hormonal contraception. Significantly decreases the effectiveness
of hormonal contraception by decreasing levonorgestrel and ethinyloestradiol
levels, most likely by inducing CYP3A4.

Main mechanisms of action

Probably similar to carbamazepine – that is, inhibition of voltage-gated sodium
channels. Both eslicarbazepine acetate and its metabolites stabilise the inacti-
vated state of voltage-gated sodium channels, preventing their return to the
activated state and thereby sustaining repetitive neuronal firing.

Pharmacokinetics

Oral bioavailability: high – the amount of metabolites recovered in urine corre-
sponded to more than 90% of an eslicarbazepine acetate dose.
Protein binding: 30%
Metabolism: Eslicarbazepine acetate is rapidly and extensively biotransformed to
its major active metabolite eslicarbazepine by hydrolytic first-pass metabolism.
Eslicarbazepine acetate metabolites are eliminated from the systemic circulation
primarily by renal excretion, in the unchanged and glucuronide conjugate forms.
Minor active metabolites in plasma are R-licarbazepine and oxcarbazepine. Esli-
carbazepine acetate does not affect its own metabolism or clearance.
Elimination half-life: 12–20 hours.

Drug interactions

Drug interactions may be significant. Eslicarbazepine acetate may have an inducing effect on the metabolism of drugs which are mainly eliminated by metabolism
through CYP3A4 (carbamazepine, phenytoin, phenobarbital, topiramate) or
conjugation through the UDP-glucuronyltransferases (lamotrigine).

> *When initiating or discontinuing treatment with eslicarbazepine acetate or
> changing the dose, it may take 2 to 3 weeks to reach the new level of enzyme
> activity. This time delay must be taken into account when eslicarbazepine
> acetate is being used just prior to or in combination with other drugs that
> require dose adjustment when co-administered with eslicarbazepine acetate.*

Also, eslicarbazepine has inhibiting properties with respect to CYP2C19 and
therefore interacts in co-medication with drugs that are mainly metabolised
by CYP2C19.
Concomitant administration of eslicarbazepine acetate with
- phenytoin significantly decreases exposure to eslicarbazepine (most
  likely caused by an induction of glucuronidation) and increases exposure to phenytoin (most likely caused by CYP2C19 inhibition)
- lamotrigine is expected to lead to interactions because glucuronidation
  is the major metabolic pathway for both of these drugs. However, their

co-administration in healthy subjects showed a minor average pharmacokinetic interaction (exposure of lamotrigine decreased 15%)
- topiramate mildly decreases exposure to topiramate (most likely caused by a reduced bioavailability of topiramate)
- carbamazepine significantly increases the risk of diplopia, ataxia and dizziness. Carbamazepine increases eslicarbazepine clearance and vice versa.

Concomitant administration with valproate or levetiracetam appeared not to affect the exposure to eslicarbazepine.

Main disadvantages

Eslicarbazepine acetate has been developed with the intention that it should have less interaction potential with other drugs than its parent drug carbamazepine and no auto-induction by preventing the formation of toxic epoxide metabolites such as carbamazepine-10,11 epoxide. However, this appears to be an unfulfilled promise because eslicarbazepine acetate has many drug interactions. Whether it will match the success of carbamazepine is too early to assess.

Ethosuximide

7

Ethosuximide (α-ethyl-α-methyl-succinimide) is the main survivor of the succinimides.[46-48] It was first introduced in clinical practice in the early 1950s for the treatment of 'petit mal'.[49]

Authorised indications

UK-SmPC: primarily useful in absence seizures. When GTCSs and other forms of epilepsy co-exist with absence seizures, ethosuximide may be administered in combination with other AEDs.
FDA-PI: control of absence (petit mal) epilepsy.

Clinical applications

Ethosuximide is still a valuable AED for the treatment of typical absence seizures and has a 70% seizure-free success rate as monotherapy.[6] It is recommended in childhood absence epilepsy (monotherapy) and IGEs with intractable absence seizures (adjunctive therapy).

   Ethosuximide is also useful as adjunctive treatment in negative myoclonus,[50] drop attacks[51] and certain types of myoclonic epilepsy.[52] An anecdotal view that ethosuximide does not control GTCS has recently been challenged.[53]

Dosage and titration

Titrate slowly to avoid ADRs, mainly gastrointestinal disturbances.
Adults and children over 12 years: start treatment with 250 mg/day and increase slowly in 250 mg increments every 4–7 days, to up to 750–1500 mg.
Children under 12 years: start with 5–10 mg/kg/day and increase slowly to 20–35 mg/kg/day.
Dosing: two or three times daily.
TDM: mostly not needed.
Reference range: 40–100 mg/l (300–700 µmol/l).

Main ADRs

Common and/or important: gastrointestinal symptoms include anorexia, vague gastric upset, nausea and vomiting, cramps, epigastric and abdominal pain and diarrhoea. Drowsiness, weight loss photophobia, euphoria, hiccups, headache and, less often, behavioural and psychotic disturbances may occur.
Serious: haemopoietic complications (aplastic anaemia), Stevens–Johnson syndrome, renal and hepatic impairment, and systemic lupus erythematosus.

Considerations in women

Pregnancy: category C.
Interaction with hormonal contraception: none.

Main mechanisms of action

Ethosuximide exerts its anti-absence effect by either reducing thalamic low threshold calcium currents, probably by a direct channel-blocking action that is voltage dependent,[54] or through a potent inhibitory effect in the perioral region of the primary somatosensory cortex.[55]

Pharmacokinetics

Oral bioavailability: 90–100%.
Protein binding: 85%.
Metabolism: hepatic oxidation and then conjugation.
Elimination half-life: 30–60 hours.

Drug interactions

Commonly, there are no clinically significant drug–drug interactions. Ethosuximide may raise the plasma concentration of phenytoin. Valproate has been reported to both increase and decrease ethosuximide levels.

Main disadvantages

- Narrow spectrum of anti-epileptic activity.
- It sometimes exhibits severe adverse idiosyncratic reactions.
- Abrupt withdrawal in patients with absences may precipitate absence status epilepticus.

Other available succinimides

Methsuximide is a broader spectrum drug than ethosuximide (but with a weaker action) and is also effective in focal seizures. ADRs are more frequent and may be more serious than with ethosuximide.
Phensuximide is rarely used because its effect is inferior to other succinimides.

Felbamate[56-59]

8

In 1993, felbamate, a 2-phenyl-1,3-propanediol dicarbamate, became the first AED since 1978 to be approved by the FDA with the brand name Felbatol. Unlike its dicarbamate analog meprobamate, it has minimal anxiolytic and sedative-hypnotic effects in therapeutic doses.

Authorised indications
UK-SmPC: not licensed.
FDA-PI: alone or as an adjunct in the treatment of focal seizures in adults and as an adjunct in focal and generalised seizures of Lennox–Gastaut syndrome in children.

> *Warnings apply: felbamate should only be used in patients who respond inadequately to alternative treatments and whose epilepsy is so severe that a substantial risk of aplastic anaemia and/ or liver failure is deemed acceptable in light of the benefits conferred by its use.*

Clinical applications
The clinical use of felbamate as an AED practically ended 1 year after its FDA approval, when it became apparent that felbamate is associated with a high incidence of aplastic anaemia and hepatic failure, and also with some fatalities. [60-63] In addition, felbamate is difficult to use because of its narrow therapeutic range and significant drug–drug interactions. Currently, the use of felbamate as an AED is cautiously limited to severe cases of Lennox–Gastaut syndrome, mainly with atonic/astatic seizures, and with bi-monthly follow-up of transaminases and blood cell counts. Possibly, the risk of using felbamate in Lennox–Gastaut syndrome outweighs any benefits, which, even if they occur, are short lived.

However, an expert panel concluded in 2006 that "although felbamate is not indicated as first-line AED, its utility in treating seizures that are refractory to other AEDs is undisputed, as shown by the number of patients who continue to use it. New exposures to felbamate number approximately 3200–4200 patients annually, and it is estimated that over the past 10 years, approximately 35,000 new starts have occurred."[57]
Author's note: The stated numbers in the above quotation cannot be used as evidence of effectiveness because they are influenced by factors other than efficacy.

Dosage and titration
Adults (14 years of age and older): start felbamate at 1200 mg/day in three or four divided doses while reducing present AEDs by 20% in order to control plasma

levels of concurrent phenytoin, valproate, phenobarbital, and carbamazepine and its metabolites. Further reductions of the concomitant AEDs dosage may be necessary to minimise side effects due to drug interactions. Titrate in increments of 1200 mg/day at weekly intervals to a maintenance dose of 3600 mg/day. Higher doses of 5000–6000 mg/day may be used. If the patient is not taking enzyme-inducing AED, then a slower titration is recommended.

Children with Lennox–Gastaut Syndrome (2–14 years of age): start felbamate at 15 mg/kg/day in three or four divided doses while reducing present AEDs by 20% in order to control plasma levels of concurrent phenytoin, valproic acid, phenobarbital, and carbamazepine and its metabolites. Further reductions of the concomitant AEDs dosage may be necessary to minimise side effects due to drug interactions. Titrate in increments of 15 mg/kg/day at weekly intervals to a maintenance dose of 45 mg/kg/day.

Dosing: Three to four times daily.

TDM: It is mandatory because of its many interactions with other AEDs.

Reference range: 50–110 mg/l (300–750 umol/l)

Main ADRs

It is because of serious ADRs that felbamate has been downgraded in its license indications and clinical practice.

Frequent and/or important: insomnia, anorexia, nausea, dizziness, headache, vomiting, weight loss, irritability, hyperactivity and behavioural disturbances.

Serious: Aplastic anaemia and hepatic failure which are usually seen during the first 6–12 months of felbamate therapy.

Aplastic anaemia: Aplastic anaemia (pancytopenia in the presence of a bone marrow largely depleted of hematopoietic precursors) occurs with felbamate at an incidence that may be more than a 100 fold greater than that seen in the untreated population (i.e., 2 to 5 per million persons per year). The risk of death in patients with aplastic anaemia generally varies as a function of its severity and aetiology; current estimates of the overall case fatality rate are in the range of 20–30%, but rates as high as 70% have been reported in the past. There are too few felbamate-associated cases, and too little known about them, to provide a reliable estimate of the syndrome's incidence or its case fatality rate or to identify the factors, if any, that might conceivably be used to predict who is at greater or lesser risk. Most of the cases of aplastic anaemia with felbamate occurred in women over the age of 17 years with a history of idiosyncratic reactions to other AEDs or a history of cytopenia, allergy and underlying autoimmune disease previous to felbamate use.[57] It was not reported in children younger than 13 years.

In managing patients on felbamate, it should be borne in mind that the clinical manifestation of aplastic anaemia may not be seen until after a patient has been on this drug from 5–30 weeks. However, the injury to bone marrow stem cells that is held to be ultimately responsible for the anaemia may occur weeks to months earlier. It is not known whether or not the risk of developing aplastic anaemia changes with duration of exposure. Consequently, it is not safe to assume that a patient who has been on felbamate without signs of haematologic abnormality for long periods of time is without risk.

It is not known whether or not the dose of felbamate or concomitant use of AEDs and/or other drugs affects the incidence of aplastic anaemia.

Aplastic anaemia typically develops without premonitory clinical or laboratory signs, the full blown syndrome presenting with signs of infection, bleeding, or anaemia. Accordingly, routine blood testing cannot be reliably used to reduce the incidence of aplastic anaemia, but it will, in some cases, allow the detection of the haematologic changes before the syndrome declares itself clinically.

Hepatic failure: this has mainly occurred in young children. The reported rate of hepatic failure with felbamate in the US has been about 6 cases leading to death or transplant per 75,000 patient years of use. This rate may be an underestimate because of under-reporting. Of the cases reported, about 67% resulted in death or liver transplantation, usually within 5 weeks of the onset of signs and symptoms of liver failure. The earliest onset of severe hepatic dysfunction followed subsequently by liver failure was 3 weeks after initiation of felbamate. Some reports described dark urine and nonspecific prodromal symptoms (e.g., anorexia, malaise, and gastrointestinal symptoms) but in other reports it was not clear if any prodromal symptoms preceded the onset of jaundice. It is not known whether or not the risk of developing hepatic failure changes with duration of exposure. It is also not known whether or not the dosage of felbamate or concomitant use of other drugs affects the incidence of hepatic failure.

It has not been proved that periodic serum transaminase testing will prevent serious hepatic injury but it is generally believed that early detection of drug-induced hepatic injury along with immediate withdrawal of the suspect drug enhances the likelihood for recovery. There is no information available that documents how rapidly patients can progress from normal liver function to liver failure, but other drugs known to be hepatotoxins can cause liver failure rapidly (e.g., from normal enzymes to liver failure in 2-4 weeks). Accordingly, monitoring of serum transaminase levels is recommended at baseline and periodically thereafter. Felbamate should be discontinued if either serum alanine or aspartate transaminase levels become increased ≥ 2 times the upper limit of normal, or if clinical signs and symptoms suggest liver failure.

> *FDA warning: All patients who are currently taking or starting on felbamate for any indication should be monitored for notable changes in behaviour that could indicate the emergence or worsening of suicidal thoughts or behaviour or depression.*

Considerations in women

Pregnancy: category C.
Breastfeeding: unknown but excreted in human breast milk.
Interactions with hormonal contraception: Significant reduction of the efficacy of hormonal contraception.

Main mechanisms of action

These are unknown and but are likely to be multiple. The most probable mechanisms are (a) potentiation of GABA responses via its interaction with a site on the $GABA_A$ receptor that is distinct from the benzodiazepine recognition site and (b) inhibition of N-methyl-D-aspartate (NMDA) receptors via a channel-blocking action and also possibly by distinct effects on channel gating.

Felbamate has weak inhibitory effects on GABA receptor binding and benzodiazepine receptor binding and is devoid of activity at the MK-801 receptor binding site of the NMDA receptor-ionophore complex. However, felbamate does interact as an antagonist at the strychnine-insensitive glycine recognition site of the NMDA receptor-ionophore complex.

Pharmacokinetics

Oral bioavailability: 90%

Protein binding: 22% to 25%

Metabolism: Felbamate is metabolised by the hepatic CYP3A4 system and it is an enzyme inhibitor. Following oral administration, about 40–50% of absorbed dose appears unchanged in urine, and an additional 40% is present as unidentified metabolites and conjugates. About 15% is present as parahydroxyfelbamate, 2-hydroxyfelbamate, and felbamate monocarbamate, none of which have significant antiepileptic activity.

Elimination half life: 20 hours (without enzyme-inducing drugs).

Drug interactions

These are numerous. Felbamate significantly increases the plasma levels of phenytoin, valproate, carbamazepine epoxide (but decreases carbamazepine) and phenobarbital. Conversely, phenytoin, carbamazepine and phenobarbital approximately double the clearance of felbamate and, therefore, their addition causes a significant decrease in the plasma levels of felbamate. Valproate probably does not affect felbamate. Felbamate's interaction with newer AEDs is not well studied, but the elimination of felbamate is strikingly reduced in co-medication with gabapentin.[64]

Main disadvantages

Probably more disadvantages than advantages.

Gabapentin

9

Gabapentin (1-[aminomethyl]-cyclohexaneacetic acid) first received marketing approval as an adjunctive AED for the treatment of focal epilepsies in 1993.[65,66]

Authorised indications

UK-SmPC: (1) monotherapy in the treatment of focal seizures with and without secondary generalisation in adults and adolescents aged 12 years and above and (2) adjunctive therapy of focal seizures with and without secondary generalisation in patients >6 years of age.

FDA-PI: (1) adjunctive therapy of focal seizures with and without secondary generalisation in patients over 12 years of age; (2) adjunctive therapy of focal seizures in children aged 3–12 years.

Clinical applications

Recommendations for gabapentin as an AED are limited to focal seizures. It is the least effective of all the other newer AEDs, even at higher doses of around 3000 mg/day.[67] However, it is considered relatively safe with few ADRs. It is mainly used for non-epileptic disorders such as neuropathic pain.

It is contraindicated for generalised-onset seizures of any type (absences, myoclonic jerks, GTCSs) because it is either ineffective or may exaggerate them.[68–70]

Dosage and titration

Adults: start with 300 mg/day and increase rapidly in increments of 300 mg/day up to a typical adult maintenance dose of 900–1800 mg/day given in three divided doses. Doses of up to 3600 mg/day have been used.

Children: start treatment with 15 mg/kg/day and increase to 30 mg/kg/day within a few days. The recommended maintenance dose is 50–100 mg/day. Children require relatively higher doses than adults, because clearance of gabapentin is greater in children than in adults.

Dosing: three times daily.

TDM: usually not needed; its dose-dependent absorption increases its pharmacokinetic variability.[71,72]

Reference range: 2–20 mg/l (12–120 µmol/l).

Main ADRs

Gabapentin has a relatively good adverse reaction profile.

Frequent and/or important: increased appetite and weight gain is a problem. Other reactions include dizziness, ataxia, nystagmus, headache, tremor, fatigue, diplopia, rhinitis and nausea. Significant behavioural disturbances, such as aggression, hyperexcitability and tantrums, have been reported, mainly in children.[73] Caution is recommended in patients with a history of psychotic illness. *Serious:* rarely, rash (0.5%), leucopenia (0.2%) and ECG changes and angina (0.05%).

Gabapentin may unmask myasthenia gravis.[74]

> *FDA warning: All patients who are currently taking or starting on gabapentin for any indication should be monitored for notable changes in behaviour that could indicate the emergence or worsening of suicidal thoughts or behaviour or depression.*

Considerations in women

Pregnancy: category C but with teratogenic effects in animal exposure.[75]
Breastfeeding: it is excreted in breast milk, but the effect on the nursing infant is unknown.
Interaction with hormonal contraception: none.
Others: weight gain may be of particular importance to women because of the associated risk for polycystic ovary syndrome.

Main mechanisms of action

The mechanism of action is uncertain. Gabapentin was developed because of its structural similarity to GABA and its ability to cross the blood–brain barrier. However, it does not appear to be a GABA agonist.

The mechanism responsible for its anti-epileptic activity and the relief of neuropathic pain is probably due to a modulating action of gabapentin on voltage-gated calcium channels and neurotransmitter release.

Pharmacokinetics

Oral bioavailability: low <60%. Gabapentin is rapidly absorbed and reaches peak plasma levels within 2–4 hours after oral ingestion. Bioavailability is less than 60%, but is dose-dependent; absorption is progressively reduced with an increasing dosage. Food intake does not influence absorption.
Protein binding: none.
Metabolism: gabapentin is not metabolised and is excreted by the kidneys in unchanged form. Renal impairment reduces drug clearance and raises plasma gabapentin concentrations.
Elimination half-life: 5–9 hours.

Drug interactions

There are no significant interactions with other AEDs. However, cimetidine reduces the renal clearance of gabapentin and antacids reduce the absorption of gabapentin by 20%.

Main disadvantages

A narrow-spectrum and low-efficiency AED that is limited to the treatment of focal seizures.

Therapeutic efficacy is weak in relation to other AEDs, the number of responders is disappointingly low even when higher doses are used and it is unusual for patients with severe focal epilepsies to derive much benefit.

Lacosamide[76-84]

10

Lacosamide is a functionalised amino acid (R)-2-acetamido-N-benzyl-3-methoxypropionamide. It is one of the latest AEDs to be licensed (at the end of 2008), under the brand name Vimpat.

Authorised indications

SmPC: adjunctive therapy in the treatment of focal seizures with or without secondary generalisation in patients with epilepsy aged 16 years and older. Solution for infusion is an alternative for patients for whom oral administration is temporarily not feasible.

FDA: (1) tablets are indicated as adjunctive therapy in the treatment of focal seizures in patients with epilepsy aged 17 years and older and (2) injection for intravenous use is indicated as adjunctive therapy in the treatment of focal seizures in patients with epilepsy aged 17 years and older when oral administration is temporarily not feasible

Clinical applications

Based on RCTs, lacosamide is a useful addition to our armamentarium in the treatment of epilepsy. This is also supported by experience since its introduction in clinical practice.

Lacosamide has proven efficacy and a high retention rate (77% in a year) in difficult to treat patients. It is particularly important in adjunctive AED therapy because of its excellent pharmacokinetic profile, minimal drug to drug interactions, good safety and novel mechanism/s of action, which is different than any other AED co-medication. It is considered as having less sedative effects than most other AEDs. Intravenous solution is important when oral drug administration is impossible.

Dosage and titration

"Start low and go slow"

Adults: Start with 50 mg twice daily (100 mg/day). Increase at weekly intervals by 100 mg/day to 200–400 mg/day.

> The maximum recommended dose of lacosamide is 400 mg/day because higher doses may be associated with CNS and gastrointestinal ADRs.

A maximum dose of 300 mg/day is recommended by the FDA for patients with mild or moderate hepatic impairment; no such upper limits are recommended by the EMEA.

Lacosamide injection (without further dilution or mixed in compatible diluents) should be administered intravenously over 15–60 min. When switching from oral lacosamide, the initial total daily intravenous dosage should be equivalent to the total daily dosage and frequency of oral lacosamide. When used as short-term replacement for oral lacosamide, intravenous lacosamide was well tolerated when administered as a 15-, 30- or 60-min infusion.
Dosing: twice daily
TDM: unknown.
Reference range: unknown.

Main ADRs

Frequent and/or important: Dizziness, headache, diplopia, nausea, vomiting and blurred vision.
Serious: A small, asymptomatic, dose-related increase in the PR interval measured on ECG has been observed in clinical studies. However, atrioventricular block is uncommon, with an occurrrence of 0.7%, 0%, 0.5% and 0% for lacosamide 200 mg, 400 mg, 600 mg or placebo, respectively. No second or higher degree atrioventricular block was seen in lacosamide patients. Also, the incidence rate for syncope did not differ between lacosamide (0.1%) and placebo treated epilepsy patients (0.3%). However, caution is needed in patients with known conduction problems or severe cardiac disease, in the elderly and in comedication with drugs known to be associated with PR prolongation (e.g. carbamazepine, lamotrigine, pregabalin, eslicarbazepine or class I antiarrhythmic drugs), though an increased magnitude of PR prolongation has not been found so far in comedication with carbamazepine or lamotrigine.

Considerations in women

Pregnancy: category C.
Breastfeeding: unknown but possibly excreted in breast milk (animal data).
Interactions with hormonal contraception: none.

Main mechanisms of action

Not fully elucidated but two mechanisms are possible: (a) lacosamide selectively enhances slow inactivation of voltage-gated sodium channels, resulting in stabilisation of hyperexcitable neuronal membranes and inhibition of repetitive neuronal firing and (b) lacosamide may bind to collapsin response mediator protein–2 (CRMP–2), a phosphoprotein which is mainly expressed in the nervous system and is involved in neuronal differentiation and control of axonal outgrowth. The role of CRMP-2 binding in seizure control is unknown.

Pharmacokinetics

Lacosamide has near-ideal pharmacokinetics (score 96 out of maximal best 100).
Oral bioavailability: 100%.
Protein binding: <15%

Metabolism: Primarily eliminated by renal excretion and biotransformation. Its metabolism has not been fully elucidated but CYP-2C19 is involved in the demethylation of lacosamide. Lacosamide showed no potential to induce or inhibit the activity of CYP isoforms 1A1, 1A2, 2A2, 2A6, 2B6, 2C8, 2C9, 2C19, 2D6, 2E1 and 3A4 in human hepatocytes at therapeutic concentrations, although inhibition of the CYP2C19 iso-enzyme was noted at concentrations 15-times higher than therapeutic concentrations.

Elimination half-life: 13 hours.

Drug interactions

These are minimal and probably of no clinical significance. From available evidence, lacosamide does not affect plasma levels of carbamazepine or its epoxide metabolite, gabapentin, lamotrigine, levetiracetam, oxcarbazepine, phenytoin, topiramate, valproate and zonisamide or the oral contraceptive levonorgestrel/ethinylestradiol, metformin and digoxin.[76] Carbamazepine, phenytoin and phenobarbital may decrease plasma levels of lacosamide by 15–20%. Omeprazole (a CYP2C19 inhibitor) did not produce any clinically significant changes in lacosamide plasma concentrations.

Main disadvantages

Not yet exposed to lengthy clinical practice but its use so far has met with favourable results.

Lamotrigine

11

Lamotrigine is a 3,5-diamino-6-(2,3-dichlorophenyl)-*as*-triazine of the phenyltriazine class. It was first licensed for clinical practice in 1991. Lamotrigine is one of the best newer AEDs, although there are now concerns for its use in women and myoclonic epilepsies.

Authorised indications

UK-SmPC: (1) Adults and adolescents aged 13 years and above: (a) adjunctive or monotherapy treatment of focal seizures and generalised seizures, including tonic clonic seizures and (b) seizures associated with Lennox–Gastaut syndrome. Lamotrigine is given as adjunctive therapy but may be the initial antiepileptic drug to start with in Lennox–Gastaut syndrome. (2) Children and adolescents aged 2 to 12 years: (a) adjunctive treatment of partial seizures and generalised seizures, including tonic clonic seizures and the seizures associated with Lennox Gastaut syndrome and (b) monotherapy of typical absence seizures.

FDA-PI: (1) adjunctive therapy for focal seizures and primarily GTSC in patients ≥2 years of age; (2) adjunctive therapy for the generalised seizures of Lennox–Gastaut syndrome; and (3) conversion to monotherapy in adults (≥16 years of age) with focal seizures who are receiving treatment with carbamazepine, phenytoin, phenobarbital, primidone or valproate as the single AED.

Safety and effectiveness of lamotrigine have not been established (1) as initial monotherapy; (2) for conversion to monotherapy from AEDs other than carbamazepine, phenytoin, phenobarbital, primidone, or valproate; or (3) for simultaneous conversion to monotherapy from two or more concomitant AEDs.

Clinical applications

Lamotrigine is an effective broad-spectrum AED for the treatment of all types of seizures except myoclonic jerks.[85–92] It has been recommended for all focal or generalised, idiopathic or symptomatic epileptic syndromes of adults,[88–90] children[85,86] and neonates.[93] Exceptions to this are syndromes with predominantly myoclonic jerks.

In monotherapy of focal seizures and primarily GTCSs, lamotrigine has less efficacy than carbamazepine but it is better tolerated.[94,95] The conclusions of a recent meta-analysis[94] and the SANAD report[65] comparing lamotrigine and carbamazepine have been debated.[96–99]

In polytherapy, lamotrigine is at its best efficacy when combined with valproate, because of beneficial pharmacodynamic interactions (increased therapeutic efficacy),[100] although it may also be detrimental (increased risk of ADRs and teratogenicity). This combination may be ideal for drug-resistant generalised epilepsies including those with myoclonic seizures.[101] Usually, small doses of lamotrigine added to valproate may render previously uncontrolled patients seizure-free.[6,100,102,103]

Other major advantages are that it lacks significant cognitive and behavioural ADRs and it is non-sedating with improved global functioning, which includes increased attention and alertness, which has been reported in both paediatric and adult trials.[87,104,105] Adjunctive lamotrigine significantly improved anger-hostility subscale scores relative to adjunctive levetiracetam in patients with focal seizures at the end of 20 weeks and similar improvement with lamotrigine versus levetiracetam was observed for other mood symptoms.[106] Idiosyncratic reactions, mainly rash, that can become very serious are a significant disadvantage.[107-109]

Exacerbation of seizures: increase in seizure frequency, mainly myoclonic jerks, has been reported in JME and Dravet syndrome.

Dosage and titration

'Start very low and go very slow' is essential in both adults and children.

Dosage and titration vary considerably between monotherapy, co-medication with valproate and co-medication with enzyme-inducing AEDs. For this reason the manufacturers have provided detailed tables to be followed in each of these circumstances in children and adults. The following are some examples:

Adults and children over 12 years (monotherapy): start with 25 mg once daily for 2 weeks, followed by 50 mg once daily for 2 weeks. Thereafter, the dose should be increased by a maximum of 50–100 mg every 1 or 2 weeks until the optimal response is achieved. The usual maintenance dose to achieve optimal response is 100–200 mg/day given once daily or as two divided doses. Some patients have required 500 mg/day to achieve the desired response.

Adults and children over 12 years (add-on therapy with valproate): start with 25 mg every alternate day for 2 weeks, followed by 25 mg once daily for 2 weeks. Thereafter, the dose should be increased by a maximum of 25–50 mg every 1 or 2 weeks until the optimal response is achieved. The usual maintenance dose to achieve optimal response is 100–200 mg/day given once daily or in two divided doses.

Adults and children over 12 years (add-on therapy with enzyme-inducing AEDs): start with 50 mg once daily for 2 weeks, followed by 100 mg/day given in two divided doses for 2 weeks. Thereafter, the dose should be increased by a maximum of 100 mg every 1 or 2 weeks until the optimal response is achieved. The usual maintenance dose to achieve optimal response is 200–400 mg/day given in two divided doses. Some patients have required 700 mg/day to achieve the desired response.

Children aged 2–12 years (with valproate co-medication): start treatment with 0.15 mg/kg given once daily for 2 weeks, followed by 0.3 mg/kg given once daily for 2 weeks. Thereafter, the dose should be increased by a maximum of 0.3

mg/kg every 1 or 2 weeks until the optimal response is achieved. The usual maintenance dose to achieve optimal response is 1–5 mg/kg given once daily or in two divided doses.

Children aged 2–12 years (co-medication with enzyme-inducing AEDs): start with 0.6 mg/kg/day given in two divided doses for 2 weeks, followed by 1.2 mg/kg/day for 2 weeks. Thereafter, the dose should be increased by a maximum of 1.2 mg/kg every 1 or 2 weeks until the optimal response is achieved. The usual maintenance dose to achieve optimal response is 5–15 mg/kg/day in two divided doses.

Cautionary note

A slower dosage titration probably reduces the risk of skin rash and possibly reduces the risk of generalised hypersensitivity reactions.[108] Therefore, it is mandatory to follow the recommendations of the manufacturers regarding initial dose and subsequent slow-dose escalation of lamotrigine.

Conversion to monotherapy from polytherapy with valproate or with enzyme-inducing AEDs should follow appropriate guidelines provided by the manufacturers of lamotrigine.

If lamotrigine has to be replaced by valproate, a satisfying outcome has been found after suddenly and completely withdrawing lamotrigine and introducing the valproate maintenance dosage rapidly.[110]

Useful note

TDM of newer AEDS that are metabolised[71,72]
For newer AEDs that are metabolised (felbamate, lamotrigine, oxcarbazepine, tiagabine and zonisamide), pharmacokinetic variability is just as relevant as for many of the older AEDs, mainly because of pronounced inter-individual variability in their pharmacokinetics.

TDM: it was not recommended initially for lamotrigine and other newer AEDs, but this has now been revised (see useful note).[71,72,111] More specifically, TDM for lamotrigine is particularly useful in pregnancy,[112–114] in conjunction with hormonal contraception[115] and post-operatively.[116]

Reference range: 1–15 mg/l (10–60 µmol/l).

Main ADRs

Common and/or important: skin rash, headache, nausea, diplopia, dizziness, ataxia, tremor, asthenia, anxiety, aggression, irritability, insomnia, somnolence, vomiting, diarrhoea, confusion, hallucinations and movement disorders.

Serious: an allergic skin rash is the most common and probably the most dangerous ADR, prompting withdrawal of lamotrigine.[108,109] Skin rash occurs in approximately 10% of patients, but serious rashes leading to hospitalisation, including Stevens–Johnson syndrome and anticonvulsant hypersensitivity syndrome, occur in approximately 1 out of 300 adults and 1 out of 100 children (<16 years of age) treated with lamotrigine.[108]

Nearly all cases of life-threatening rashes associated with lamotrigine have occurred within 2–8 weeks of treatment initiation. However, isolated cases have been reported after prolonged treatment (e.g. 6 months). Accordingly, duration of therapy cannot be relied on as a means to predict the potential risk heralded by the first appearance of a rash.

There are suggestions, still to be proven, that the risk of rash may also be increased by: (1) the co-administration of lamotrigine with valproate; (2) exceeding the recommended initial dose of lamotrigine; or (3) exceeding the recommended dose escalation for lamotrigine. However, cases have been reported in the absence of these factors. The incidence of skin rash can probably be reduced by starting treatment with a low dose spread over longer intervals, particularly in patients receiving concomitant valproate, which inhibits lamotrigine metabolism.

Although benign rashes also occur with lamotrigine, it is not possible to predict reliably which rashes will prove to be serious or life threatening. Accordingly, lamotrigine should ordinarily be discontinued at the first sign of rash, unless the rash is clearly not drug related. Discontinuation of treatment may not prevent a rash from becoming life threatening, or permanently disabling or disfiguring.

Patients should be advised to immediately report any symptoms of skin rash, hives, fever, swollen lymph glands, painful sores in the mouth or around the eyes, or swelling of lips or tongue, because these symptoms may be the first signs of a serious reaction.

Cardiac arrhythmia and sudden unexpected death (SUDEP): a recent report described SUDEP of four women with IGE treated with lamotrigine mono-therapy.[117] Lamotrigine inhibits the cardiac rapid delayed rectifier potassium ion current (I_{Kr}). I_{Kr}-blocking drugs may increase the risk of cardiac arrhythmia and SUDEP. The authors of the report called for a systematic study to assess whether lamotrigine may increase the risk of SUDEP in certain groups of patients[117], which generated an interesting exchange of views.[118,119] In the SANAD study, four of ten deaths related to epilepsy occurred in patients treated with lamotrigine, three with oxcarbazepine, two with gabapentin, one with carbamazepine and none with topiramate.[95] A recent study found that therapeutic doses of lamotrigine (100–400 mg daily) were not associated with QT prolongation in healthy subjects.[120] Also, clinically significant ECG changes were not common during treatment with either lamotrigine or carbamazepine in elderly patients with no pre-existing significant AV conduction defects.[121]

Other potentially serious ADRs: there have been reports of haematological abnormalities, which may or may not be associated with anticonvulsant hypersensitivity syndrome. These have included neutropenia, leucopenia, anaemia, thrombo-cytopenia, pancytopenia and, very rarely, aplastic anaemia and agranulocytosis. Elevations of liver function tests and rare reports of hepatic dysfunction, including hepatic failure, have been reported. Hepatic dysfunction usually occurs in association with hypersensitivity reactions, but isolated cases have been reported without overt signs of hypersensitivity.

Very rarely, lupus-like reactions have been reported.

> *FDA warning: All patients who are currently taking or starting on lamotrigine for any indication should be monitored for notable changes in behaviour that could indicate the emergence or worsening of suicidal thoughts or behaviour or depression.*

Considerations in women

Pregnancy: category C. However, there is recent evidence of teratogenicity that resulted in lamotrigine being downgraded to category D in the Australian PI. For example, an increased risk for non-syndromic cleft palate among infants exposed to lamotrigine during pregnancy[122] (not replicated in other pregnancy registries)[123] and a dose-related effect with MCMs have been reported.[17] The risk for MCMs in women on a combination of lamotrigine with valproate is around 10%.[17,124]

Breastfeeding: significant amounts of lamotrigine (40–60%) are excreted in breast milk. In breast-fed infants, plasma concentrations of lamotrigine reached levels at which pharmacological effects may occur.

Interactions with oral hormonal contraception and pregnancy: oral contraceptives are not significantly affected by lamotrigine, though a modest increase in levonorgestrel clearance is observed. However, pregnancy[112–114,125] and hormonal contraception[115,126] significantly lower lamotrigine levels (by more than half). Patients may suffer breakthrough seizures, mainly during the first trimester of pregnancy (if lamotrigine levels are not corrected) or toxic effects postpartum (if lamotrigine levels are adjusted during pregnancy, but not after delivery). Gradual transient increases in lamotrigine levels will occur during the week of no active hormone preparation (pill-free week).

Liver function tests should probably be monitored in infants of lamotrigine-treated mothers, as γ-glutamyl transpeptidase enzyme elevation might suggest liver damage.[127]

Main mechanisms of action

The precise mechanisms by which lamotrigine exerts its anti-epileptic action are unknown. The most likely mechanism is inhibition of voltage-gated sodium channels, thereby stabilising neuronal membranes and consequently modulating presynaptic transmitter release of excitatory amino acids (e.g. glutamate and aspartate).

Pharmacokinetics

Oral bioavailability: <100%. Lamotrigine is rapidly and completely absorbed from the gut with no significant first-pass metabolism.

Protein binding: 55%.

Metabolism: lamotrigine is predominantly metabolised in the liver by glucuronic acid conjugation. UGT1A4 is the main enzyme responsible for N-glucuronidation of lamotrigine. The major metabolite is an inactive 2-N-glucuronide conjugate. Lamotrigine is a weak UGT enzyme inducer.

Elimination half-life: 29 hours, but this is greatly affected by concomitant medication. Mean half-life is reduced to approximately 14 hours when given with enzyme-inducing drugs and is increased to a mean of approximately 70 hours when co-administered with valproate alone. Valproate is a potent inhibitor of UGT-dependent metabolism of lamotrigine, while enzyme-inducer AEDs are potent inducers of UGT-dependent metabolism of lamotrigine, which is the reason for different schemes of lamotrigine dosage and titration when combined with these AEDs.

Furthermore, the half-life of lamotrigine is generally shorter in children than in adults, with a mean value of approximately 7 hours when given with enzyme-inducing drugs and increasing to mean values of 45–50 hours when co-administered with valproate alone.

Drug interactions

The metabolism of lamotrigine is badly affected by concomitant AEDs, which makes its use in polytherapy problematic:

- Valproate inhibits the metabolism of lamotrigine, doubling or tripling its half-life,[107] whether given with or without carbamazepine, phenytoin, phenobarbital or primidone. Also, valproate seems to reduce the induction of lamotrigine metabolism associated with pregnancy or use of contraceptives.[125]
- Enzyme inducers, such as carbamazepine, phenytoin and phenobarbital, accelerate its elimination, but lamotrigine itself has no effect on hepatic metabolic processes.[128]

When lamotrigine is added to carbamazepine, symptoms of carbamazepine neurotoxicity (headache, diplopia, ataxia) may occur (probably because of pharmacodynamic interactions rather than elevated carbamazepine epoxide levels); this necessitates a reduction in the carbamazepine dose when lamotrigine is introduced.

Oxcarbazepine and levetiracetam do not affect the clearance of lamotrigine.

Main disadvantages

- High incidence of idiosyncratic ADRs, which, exceptionally, may be fatal.
- Very slow titration.
- Significant interactions with other AEDs requiring complex schemes of dosage and titration.
- Frequent TDM and dosage adjustments before, during and after pregnancy[112–114,125] and hormonal contraception.[115,125,129] Risk for seizure deterioration in pregnancy.

- Pro-myoclonic effect in syndromes with predominant myoclonic jerks, such as JME,[130–132] Dravet syndrome[133,134] and progressive myoclonic epilepsies.[135]

Useful clinical notes

- Recent evidence of teratogenicity and interaction with pregnancy and hormonal contraception contradict the previous promotion of lamotrigine as a female-friendly AED.
- Lamotrigine demands significant clinical attention in polytherapy, hormonal contraception and pregnancy.
- Lamotrigine also has significant pharmacodynamic interactions with valproate.
- The use of lamotrigine should follow the manufacturer's recommendations regarding titration and include a proper warning to the patient or guardians for immediate medical attention if suspicious rashes appear, unless the rash is clearly not drug related.

Levetiracetam

12

Levetiracetam is a single enantiomer, (S)-α-ethyl-2-oxo-pyrrolidine acetamide. Levetiracetam, licensed in 1999, is probably the best of all the newer AEDs.[136–144] It is chemically unrelated to any of the other current AEDs.

Authorised indications

EMEA-SmPC: (1) monotherapy in the treatment of partial onset seizures with or without secondary generalisation in patients from 16 years of age with newly diagnosed epilepsy; (2) adjunctive therapy (a) in the treatment of partial onset seizures with or without secondary generalisation in adults, children and infants from 1 month of age with epilepsy (the concentrate for solution for infusion is indicated for adults, adolescents and children from 4 years of age), (b) in the treatment of myoclonic seizures in adults and adolescents from 12 years of age with JME, and (c) in the treatment of primary generalised tonic-clonic seizures in adults and adolescents from 12 years of age with IGE.

Levetiracetam concentrate is an alternative for patients when oral administration is temporarily not feasible.

FDA-PI: (1) adjunctive therapy in the treatment of partial onset seizures in adults and children 4 years of age and older with epilepsy; (2) adjunctive therapy in the treatment of myoclonic seizures in adults and adolescents 12 years of age and older with juvenile myoclonic epilepsy; and (3) adjunctive therapy in the treatment of primary generalised tonic-clonic seizures in adults and children 6 years of age and older with idiopathic generalised epilepsy.

Levetiracetam injection is an alternative for adult patients (16 years and older) when oral administration is temporarily not feasible.

Clinical applications

Levetiracetam is probably a major breakthrough in the treatment of epilepsies, similar to that of carbamazepine and valproate in the 1960s. It is a highly effective, broad-spectrum, newer class of AED with a unique mechanism of action, and can be used to treat all focal or generalised, idiopathic or symptomatic epileptic syndromes in all age groups.

Levetiracetam is the first-choice AED in monotherapy and polytherapy of focal epilepsies, where it is the main challenger of carbamazepine. It is also the likely candidate to replace valproate in the treatment of JME and IGEs in general.

The main advantages of levetiracetam include the following:
- it is broad spectrum, which is of practical significance, particularly for clinicians who may not have special expertise in differentiating between focal and generalised epileptic seizures

- it has a relatively good safety profile[145–147] and does not cause significant idiosyncratic reactions or other serious ADRs
- it has superior pharmacokinetics (96% versus 100% of perfect score)[148]
- it does not need slow titration, the starting dose is often therapeutic for all forms of seizures and epilepsies (including the difficult-to-treat myoclonic seizures);[149] its action starts 2 days after drug initiation[150]
- it does not need laboratory tests (such as routine TDM or blood screening for ADRs)
- it is easier to use if polytherapy is necessitated (a lack of clinically significant drug–drug interactions[18,151] and a novel mechanism of action)
- it does not interact with hormonal contraception and is a pregnancy category C drug
- it does not interfere with liver function (a major problem with most other AEDs that are metabolised in the liver).

Levetiracetam has a significant and sustained proven efficacy for newly diagnosed or intractable focal seizures with or without secondary generalisation.[152–162] Addition of levetiracetam to standard medication seems to have a positive impact on health-related quality of life.[145]

Its effectiveness in generalised epileptic seizures and at any age has been documented in experimental and observational studies, postmarketing experience and RCTs. This includes IGE, JME, myoclonus and photosensitivity.[163–167]

Levetiracetam is the only one of the newer AEDs to have been successfully submitted to a prospective RCT in JME and other IGEs with myoclonic jerks. The study concluded that 'levetiracetam proved to be highly efficacious in the treatment of refractory patients with IGE experiencing myoclonic seizures. Levetiracetam's outstanding tolerability profile was also confirmed.'[163]

Its efficacy on primarily GTCSs has also been documented with RCTs.[164] That levetiracetam is a first-class AED in syndromes of IGEs has also been more recently confirmed.[165–167]

Levetiracetam also appears effective in benign childhood focal epilepsies,[168–170] as well as epileptic encephalopathies such as Lennox–Gastaut,[171,172] Landau–Kleffner[173] syndrome and myoclonic syndromes.[174]

As expected by its favourable pharmacokinetic profile, levetiracetam was found to be effective, well tolerated and safe in patients with epilepsy and other concomitant medical conditions, including brain tumours.[175,176] Considering also its relatively safe profile, levetiracetam may be a first-choice AED in the elderly.[177,178]

Levetiracetam is available in oral and intravenous formulations. Parenteral formulations are needed when oral administration is temporarily not feasible.[179]

Dosage and titration

Adults: start treatment with 1000 mg/day (twice-daily dosing), which may be sufficient for seizure control. If needed, levetiracetam can be titrated in steps of 500 mg/week to a maximum of 3000 mg/day. Personally, I recommend starting with 250 mg twice daily and titrating upwards according to the response.

Children: start with 5–10 mg/kg/day, which may be sufficient for seizure control. If needed, levetiracetam can be titrated in steps of 5–10 mg/kg/week to a usual maintenance dose of 20–40 mg/kg/day (a maximum of 60 mg/kg/day has been used) given in two equally divided doses.[137,180–183]

Based on weight, the maintenance dose for children should be 30–40% higher than that for adults. The reason for this is that levetiracetam clearance in children is 30–40% higher than in adults.[184,185] The increase, compared with adults, is even higher in infants.[186,187]

Levetiracetam administered by intravenous infusion at dosages and/or infusion rates higher than those proposed are well tolerated in healthy subjects, and the pharmacokinetic profile is consistent with that for oral levetiracetam.[188,189]

Dosing: twice daily. Dose adjustment is required for patients with renal dysfunction, but not for patients with liver disease.

TDM: usually not needed and can be efficacious from the starting dose. However, pregnancy appears to enhance the elimination of levetiracetam, resulting in a marked decline in plasma concentration, which suggests that TDM may be of value.[190]

Reference range: 6–20 mg/l (35–120 μmol/l).

Main ADRs

Levetiracetam is probably the AED that is most free from ADRs. Few major ADRs were reported in the clinical trials and, overall, their incidence in the levetiracetam-treated groups was little higher than that in the placebo groups.[191]

Frequent and/or important: the most common ADRs are somnolence, asthenia and dizziness, which are dose-dependent and reversible. Others include headache, infection (common cold or upper respiratory infections, which were not preceded by low neutrophil counts that might suggest impaired immunological status), anorexia, behavioural disturbances, pharyngitis and pain. No withdrawal-related behavioural ADRs were reported during the cross-titration period.[136,137] Levetiracetam interferes with rapid motor learning in humans due to suppression of excitatory activity in the motor cortex.[192]

Caution should be exercised when administering levetiracetam to individuals who may be prone to psychotic or psychiatric reactions.

In an uncontrolled study, add-on levetiracetam was associated with a paradoxical increase in seizure frequency, particularly in mentally retarded patients and those with difficult-to-treat focal-onset seizures treated with high doses of levetiracetam.[193] This may be avoided by using a lower initial dose and a slower dose escalation than recommended.

> *FDA warning: All patients who are currently taking or starting on levetiracetam for any indication should be monitored for notable changes in behaviour that could indicate the emergence or worsening of suicidal thoughts or behaviour or depression.*

Considerations in women

Pregnancy: category C. Recently, in the UK Epilepsy and Pregnancy Register of 117 pregnancies exposed to levetiracetam (39 in monotherapy and 78 in combination with at least one other AED), only three infants (all in the polytherapy group) had a MCM (2.7%; 95% confidence interval [CI], 0.9–7.7%).[194]

Breastfeeding: there is an extensive transfer of levetiracetam from mother to foetus and into breast milk. However, breast-fed infants have very-low levetiracetam plasma concentrations, suggesting a rapid elimination of levetiracetam.[190,195]

Interaction with hormonal contraception: none.

Main mechanisms of action

It has a novel mechanism of action that is distinct from that of other AEDs by targeting a synaptic vesicle protein in presynaptic terminals.[196–198] Its anti-epileptic activity does not involve a direct interaction with any of the three main mechanisms of the other AEDs. Thus, levetiracetam does not modulate Na$^+$ and low voltage-gated (T-type) Ca^{2+} currents, and does not induce any conventional facilitation of the GABAergic system. In contrast, levetiracetam has been observed to exert several atypical electrophysiological actions, including a moderate inhibition of high voltage-gated N-type Ca^{2+} currents, reduction of intracellular Ca^{2+} release from the endoplasmic reticulum, as well as suppression of the inhibitory effect of zinc and other negative allosteric modulators of both GABA- and glycine-gated currents.

The apparent absence of any direct interaction with conventional mechanisms involved in the action of other AEDs parallels the discovery of a specific binding site for levetiracetam. Recent experiments have shown that the synaptic vesicle protein 2A (SV2A) is the binding site of levetiracetam.[199,200]

Studies in mice lacking SV2A indicate that this protein has a crucial role in the regulation of vesicle function, probably involving a modulation of vesicle fusion. These mice seem normal at birth, but develop unusually severe seizures by 1 or 2 weeks of age and die within 3 weeks after birth.[199] Brain membranes and purified synaptic vesicles from mice lacking SV2A did not bind a tritiated derivative of levetiracetam, indicating that SV2A is necessary for levetiracetam binding. Levetiracetam and related derivatives bind to SV2A, but not to the related isoforms SV2B and SV2C expressed in fibroblasts, indicating that SV2A is sufficient for levetiracetam binding. In contrast, none of the other AEDs tested revealed any binding to SV2A.[199]

The severe seizures observed in mice lacking SV2A support the interpretation that this protein influences mechanisms of seizure generation or propagation. Furthermore, there is a strong correlation between the binding affinity of a series of levetiracetam derivatives such as brivaracetam and their anticonvulsant potency in the audiogenic seizure mice model. These results suggest that levetiracetam's interaction with SV2A provides a significant contribution to its anti-epileptic activity.

Pharmacokinetics

The pharmacokinetic profile of levetiracetam closely approximates the ideal characteristics expected of an AED, with good bioavailability, rapid achievement of steady-state concentrations, linear and time-invariant kinetics, minimal protein binding, and minimal metabolism.[201]

Levetiracetam comes especially close to fulfilling the desirable pharmacokinetic characteristics for an AED: (1) it has a high oral bioavailability, which is unaffected by food; (2) it is not significantly bound to plasma proteins; (3) it is eliminated partly in unchanged form by the kidneys and partly by hydrolysis to an inactive metabolite, without involvement of oxidative and conjugative enzymes; (4) it has linear kinetics; and (5) it is not vulnerable to important drug interactions, nor does it cause clinically significant alterations in the kinetics of concomitantly administered drugs. Although its half-life is relatively short (6–8 hours), its duration of action is longer than anticipated from its pharmacokinetics in plasma, and a twice-daily dosing regimen is adequate to produce the desired response.[151]

Oral bioavailability: 100% and it is unaffected by food. Levetiracetam is rapidly and almost completely absorbed after oral administration with peak plasma concentrations occurring in about 1 hour. The pharmacokinetics are linear and time-invariant, with low intra- and inter-subject variability.

Protein binding: <10%. Levetiracetam is not appreciably protein-bound nor does it affect the protein binding of other drugs. Its volume of distribution is close to the volume of intracellular and extracellular water.

Metabolism/elimination: the major metabolic pathway of levetiracetam (24% of dose) is an enzymatic hydrolysis of the acetamide group. This is not dependent on the hepatic CYP system. Further, levetiracetam does not inhibit or induce hepatic enzymes to produce clinically relevant interactions. Levetiracetam is eliminated from the systemic circulation by renal excretion as an unchanged drug, which represents 66% of the administered dose. The mechanism of excretion is glomerular filtration with subsequent partial tubular reabsorption. The metabolites have no known pharmacological activity and are also renally excreted.

Elimination half-life: 6–8 hours. It is shorter in children and longer in the elderly and subjects with renal impairment.

Drug interactions

Unlike the majority of other AEDs, levetiracetam has no clinically meaningful drug–drug interactions.

Other AEDs: levetiracetam does not influence the plasma concentration of existing AEDs. In addition, levetiracetam does not affect the *in vitro* glucuronidation of valproate. Enzyme inducers may decrease levetiracetam plasma levels by 20–30%.[202]

Other non-AEDs: levetiracetam has no known interactions with other drugs such as oral contraceptives, warfarin and digoxin. It does not reduce the effectiveness of oral contraceptives.

Main disadvantages

There are some reports of increased behavioural and psychiatric abnormalities, particularly in children or patients that may be prone to such problems.[203–206] An explanation for this may be the fast titration recommended by the manufacturers. A recent short-term study found that add-on levetiracetam in patients with intractable focal epilepsies has a favourable neuropsychological and psychiatric impact.[207]

Oxcarbazepine

13

Oxcarbazepine (10,11-dihydro-10-oxo-5H-dibenz[b,f]azepine-5-carboxamide) is a 0-keto derivative of carbamazepine, but these two AEDs have some significant differences.[208] The anti-epileptic activity is mainly exerted via its major metabolite, hydroxy-10,11-dihydro-5H-dibenzazepine-5-carboxamide (MHD). It was first licensed as an AED in 1990 in Denmark.

Authorised indications

UK-SmPC: monotherapy or adjunctive therapy for focal seizures with or without secondarily GTCSs in patients ≥6 years of age.
FDA-PI: (1) monotherapy or adjunctive therapy in the treatment of focal seizures in adults and as monotherapy in the treatment of focal seizures in children aged 4 years and above with epilepsy, and (2) as adjunctive therapy in children aged 2 years and above with epilepsy.

Note

Oxcarbazepine versus carbamazepine

Oxcarbazepine is similar to carbamazepine in its anti-epileptic efficacy and main mechanisms of action. However, it is better tolerated and has fewer interactions with other drugs because it does not undergo metabolism to 10,11–epoxide. In contrast to carbamazepine, involvement of the hepatic CYP-dependent enzymes in the metabolism of oxcarbazepine is minimal. Oxcarbazepine has a lower incidence of idiosyncratic reactions than carbamazepine; but hyponatraemia is more common with oxcarbazepine than carbamazepine.

The profile of oxcarbazepine is more similar to that of the slow-release carbamazepine preparations.

Clinical applications

Oxcarbazepine is a first class AED for monotherapy, conversion to monotherapy or adjunctive therapy for all types of focal seizures with or without secondarily GTCSs.[209–211] This has been documented in a series of clinical trials and by extensive clinical use. In 2003, it became the first AED to be approved by the FDA in 25 years for use as monotherapy in children with focal epilepsy.

Dosage and titration

Adults: start treatment with 150 mg/day and increase by 150 mg/day every second day until a target dose of 900–1200 mg/day is reached. Others start with

C.P. Panayiotopoulos, *Antiepileptic Drugs, Pharmacopoeia,*
© Springer-Verlag London Limited 2011

600 mg/day and increase weekly in 600 mg increments until a maintenance dose of between 1200 and 2400 mg/day is reached. I would recommend the principle of 'start low and go slow' to avoid ADRs and particularly rash.

In patients with impaired renal function (creatinine clearance <30 ml/min), oxcarbazepine should be initiated at one-half of the usual starting dose and increased slowly until the desired clinical response is achieved or ADRs appear.
Children: start with 10 mg/kg/day in two or three divided doses. The dosage can be increased by 10 mg/kg/day at approximately weekly intervals to a maximum of 30–46 mg/kg/day.
Dosing: twice or three times daily.
TDM: because of striking pharmacokinetic changes, and clinical response, oxycarbazepine levels should be monitored throughout pregnancy and the puerperium.[212,213]
Reference range: MHD, 4–12 mg/l (50–140 µmol/l).

Main ADRs

Frequent and/or important: the most common CNS adverse events are headache, dizziness, fatigue, nausea, somnolence, ataxia and diplopia. Most of these are dose related, they usually occur at the start of therapy and subside during the course of therapy.
Serious: the reported rate of skin rash with oxcarbazepine is around 2% (adults) and 5% (children), as opposed to 5–10% with carbamazepine. Multi-organ hypersensitivity disorder and Stevens–Johnson syndrome have been reported.

> *Cross-reactivity with carbamazepine is approximately 25% (i.e. of the patients who have skin rash with carbamazepine, 25% will also have skin rash with oxcarbazepine). Therefore, given the availability of other AEDs, oxcarbazepine may not be a good option for patients who developed idiosyncratic reactions with carbamazepine or other AEDs (e.g. lamotrigine and phenytoin).*

Hyponatraemia (serum sodium level <125 mmol/l) occurs in 3% of patients on oxcarbazepine. This develops gradually during the first few months of treatment. It is usually benign and can be reversed by fluid restriction or a reduction in the dose of oxcarbazepine. Acute water intoxication is rare. Measurement of serum sodium levels are needed for patients with renal disease, those taking medication that may lower serum sodium levels (e.g. diuretics, oral contra-ceptives or non-steroidal anti-inflammatory drugs) or if clinical symptoms of hyponatraemia develop.

Consumption of large volumes of any fluid should be discouraged.

Oxcarbazepine is contraindicated in patients with a history of atrio-ventricular block.

> *FDA warning: All patients who are currently taking or starting on oxcarbazepine for any indication should be monitored for notable changes in behaviour that could indicate the emergence or worsening of suicidal thoughts or behaviour or depression.*

Considerations in women

Pregnancy: category C. Seizure control may be lost during pregnancy in women on oxcarbazepine.[129] The concentration of oxcarbazepine and its metabolite decrease markedly during pregnancy and may increase several fold after delivery.[212,213]
Breastfeeding: oxcarbazepine and its active metabolite are secreted in significant amounts in breast milk.
Interaction with hormonal contraception: yes.

Main mechanisms of action

Oxcarbazepine exerts its anti-epileptic activity primarily through its major metabolite MHD. Like carbamazepine, blockade of voltage-sensitive sodium channels is its main mechanism of action. Others include reduction of the release of excitatory amino acids, probably by inhibiting high voltage-activated calcium currents. An effect on potassium channels might be clinically important.

Pharmacokinetics

Oral bioavailability: >95% and peak concentrations are reached within 4–6 hours. Absorption is unaffected by food.
Protein binding: only 38% of the MHD is bound to serum proteins, as compared with 67% for the parent compound.
Metabolism: oxcarbazepine is rapidly metabolised in the liver to form the pharmacologically active MHD. This is then conjugated to a glucuronide compound and excreted in the urine as a monohydroxy derivative.
Elimination half-life: 8–10 hours. This is shorter in children and longer in the elderly.
  As a neutral lipophilic substance, the active metabolite MHD of oxcarbazepine is able to diffuse rapidly through the various membranes and the blood–brain barrier.

Drug interactions

The oxcarbazepine–MHD complex lowers plasma concentrations of some drugs, such as hormonal contraceptives and lamotrigine, and increases the plasma concentration of others, such as phenytoin. Conversely, strong inducers of the CYP enzyme system, such as carbamazepine and phenytoin, lower plasma levels of MHD by 29–40%.
  Combination therapy with monoamine oxidase inhibitors should be avoided, because oxcarbazepine has structural similarities with tricyclic antidepressants.

Main disadvantages

- Oxcarbazepine is contraindicated in generalised seizures, such as absences or myoclonic jerks in syndromes of IGE.[214] It may not be effective in neonates and children <2 years of age.
- One out of four patients have cross sensitivity to idiosyncratic reactions with carbamazepine or other AEDs.

- Although it is among the first-choice AEDs for monotherapy in focal epilepsies, its use as polytherapy is less satisfactory because of drug–drug interactions.
- Unless levels of oxcarbazepine are adjusted, seizures may increase during pregnancy and toxicity may appear postpartum.

Useful clinical notes

- Conversion to oxcarbazepine from carbamazepine or phenytoin is complicated by the initial need for higher doses of oxcarbazepine than needed later as monotherapy.
- A carbamazepine dose of 200 mg appears to be equivalent to 300 mg of oxcarbazepine.
- It is possible to change from carbamazepine to oxcarbazepine abruptly, using a dose ratio of 200 mg carbamazepine to 300 mg oxcarbazepine, without the need for titration.[215] A lower ratio 1:1 or 1:1.25 is usually better tolerated, especially if the conversion is from slow-release preparations of carbamazepine. Levels of concomitant medication may be affected by the removal of the enzyme-inducing effects of carbamazepine.

Phenobarbital

14

Phenobarbital was introduced into clinical practice in 1912[49] and is still a widely used AED, particularly when cost is a problem.[216-219] It is highly effective in all seizure types except absences.[216-219]

Authorised indications

UK-BNF for Children: all forms of epilepsy except absence seizures in patients of any age, including neonates.
USA: focal seizures and GTCSs in patients of any age, including neonates.

Current main applications

Phenobarbital is still a main AED for neonatal and febrile seizures (if treatment is needed) and established convulsive status epilepticus. It is the main monotherapy AED in resource-poor countries.

In small doses at night, phenobarbital is useful as adjunctive therapy in many forms of epilepsies other than absences. It is still used in some European countries in the treatment of JME.

Dosage and titration

'Start very low and go very slow' is particularly important.
Maintenance dose: adults 50–200 mg at night (initial 30 mg/day) and children 3–5 mg/kg/day.
Dosing: once daily prior to going to sleep.
TDM: necessary.
Reference range: 10–40 mg/l (43–172 μmol/l).

Main ADRs

Frequent and/or important: the most common CNS adverse events are drowsiness, sedation or aggression, depression, behavioural disturbances and impairment of cognition and concentration. Hyperkinesia (hyperactivity) is a major problem in children.
Serious: hepatitis, cholestasis, thrombocytopenia, agranulocytosis; skin rash and multi-organ hypersensitivity disorder and Stevens–Johnson syndrome.

Considerations in women

Pregnancy: category D.
Breastfeeding: phenobarbital is secreted in significant amounts in breast milk (40% of the plasma concentration) and may cause sedation to the baby. However, avoiding breastfeeding may cause withdrawal symptoms to the neonate.
Interaction with hormonal contraception: yes.

Main mechanisms of action

Phenobarbital exerts its anti-epileptic activity through multiple modes of action. Its primary effect is probably through its post-synaptic binding to $GABA_A$ receptors. It also blocks voltage-sensitive sodium and potassium channels, reduces presynaptic calcium influx and possibly inhibits glutamate-mediated currents.

Pharmacokinetics

Oral bioavailability: >90% and peak concentrations are reached within 8–12 hours.
Protein binding: 20–50%.
Metabolism: phenobarbital is metabolised in the liver, mainly through hydroxylation and glucuronidation, and induces most isozymes of the CYP system.
Elimination half-life: 2–7 days. It is a very long-acting barbiturate.

Drug interactions

Phenobarbital, a potent enzyme inducer (CYP2C, CYP3A, microsomal epoxide hydrolases and UGTs), has marked and clinically significant interactions with other drugs including AEDs and hormonal contraception. It lowers the plasma concentration of carbamazepine, clonazepam, lamotrigine, phenytoin (but may also raise phenytoin concentration), tiagabine, valproate and zonisamide. Plasma levels of phenobarbital decrease in co-medication with enzyme inducers; they increase with valproate, felbamate and dextropropoxyphene.

Main disadvantages

ADRs are the main disadvantage of phenobarbital. It is primarily unsuitable for children and elderly patients.

Useful clinical notes

- It is erroneous to attempt substitution of phenobarbital in well-controlled patients unless it is associated with unacceptable ADRs.
- Withdrawal should be in very small dosages and at long intervals because of the risk of withdrawal seizures.
- Always start and titrate slowly with small doses at night (20–30 mg). Avoid high doses (maximum in adults 200 mg).

Other available main barbiturate agents

Primidone probably has similar ADRs to phenobarbital and is of no better efficacy. *UK-SmPC:* management of grand mal and psychomotor (temporal lobe) epilepsy. It is also of value in the management of focal and jacksonian seizures, myoclonic jerks and akinetic attacks.
FDA-PI: sole or adjunctive therapy in the control of grand mal, psychomotor and focal epileptic seizures in adults and children. It may control grand mal seizures refractory to other anticonvulsant therapy.
Barbexaclone is of similar effectiveness as phenobarbital, but less sedative.[221]

Phenytoin

15

Phenytoin was introduced into clinical practice in 1938[49] and is probably the most widely used AED.[222] It is highly effective in focal seizures and GTCSs.[216-218,220] It is contraindicated in absences and myoclonic jerks, progressive myoclonic epilepsies such as Unverricht syndrome, and probably in Lennox–Gastaut syndrome and other childhood epileptic encephalopathies (but may be effective in tonic seizures).

Authorised indications

UK-SmPC: control of tonic-clonic seizures (grand mal epilepsy), partial seizures (focal including temporal lobe) or a combination of these, and the prevention and treatment of seizures occurring during or following neurosurgery and/or severe head injury.

FDA-PI: control of generalised tonic-clonic (grand mal) and complex partial (psychomotor, temporal lobe) seizures and prevention and treatment of seizures occurring during or following neurosurgery.

Clinical applications

Phenytoin is still very useful in neonatal seizures (if phenobarbital fails), focal seizures and GTCSs (no other AED had superior efficacy than phenytoin in RCTs, but ADRs are hindering its use), and established convulsive or focal status epilepticus (often considered as the first choice).

Dosage and titration

Maintenance dose: adults 200–400 mg nocte (initially 50–100 mg/day) and children 5–10 mg/kg/day.

Dosing: once daily.

TDM: necessary, mainly because of its narrow therapeutic range and saturable kinetics (see metabolism).

Reference range: 10–20 mg/l (40–80 µmol/l).

Main ADRs

Serious early non-dose related: anticonvulsant hypersensitivity syndrome that may be fatal (Stevens–Johnson and Lyll's syndrome).

Dose-related: ataxia, drowsiness, lethargy, sedation and encephalopathy.

Chronic use: gingival hyperplasia, hirsutism and dysmorphism.

Other reactions: haematological, neurological (e.g. peripheral neuropathy and cerebellar atrophy) and others, such as systemic lupus erythematosus. Its effect on cognition is probably similar to that of carbamazepine, but much better than that of phenobarbital.

Considerations in women

Pregnancy: category D.
Breastfeeding: small amounts are excreted in breast milk.
Interaction with hormonal contraception: yes.

Main mechanisms of action

Blockade of voltage-sensitive sodium channels is the main mechanism of action of phenytoin.

Pharmacokinetics

Oral bioavailability: 95% and peak concentrations are reached within 4–12 hours. Absorption may be erratic; food and small bowel disease significantly alter its absorption.
Protein binding: >85%.
Metabolism: phenytoin is metabolised in the liver, mainly through para-hydroxylation by the hepatic P450 system. Its metabolism is dose-dependent because of hepatic enzyme saturation kinetics. At higher drug concentrations, phenytoin kinetics are non-linear and thus a small increase in dose may lead to a large increase in drug concentration as elimination becomes saturated.
Elimination half-life: 7–40 hours. This is plasma level and co-medication. It is shorter in children and longer in the elderly.

Drug interactions

These are multiple. Phenytoin, an enzyme inducer, significantly affects plasma levels of other drugs, including AEDs and hormonal contraception, and *vice versa*. It lowers the plasma concentration of clonazepam, carbamazepine, lamotrigine, tiagabine, topiramate, valproate, zonisamide and the active metabolite of oxcarbazepine. It often raises the plasma concentration of phenobarbital and sometimes lowers the plasma concentration of ethosuximide and primidone (by increasing conversion to phenobarbital).

Disadvantages

- Acute and long-term ADRs hamper its use.
- Long-term use of phenytoin is unsuitable for women because of aesthetic reasons and teratogenic properties.
- Therapeutic range is narrow and close to the toxic range requiring frequent monitoring of plasma levels. After a certain dose (100–200 mg/day), further increases should be small (25 mg/day) and over longer intervals (every 2–4 weeks).

Useful clinical notes

Phenytoin is a very effective drug in focal seizures and secondarily GTCSs, but it is often contraindicated in generalised epilepsies.

Other available phenytoin-related agents

Phosphenytoin for intramuscular and intravenous use; it is preferred to phenytoin because it does not produce adverse tissue effects.[223–228]

Ethotoin and mephenytoin probably offer no advantage over phenytoin.

Pregabalin

16

Pregabalin [(S)-3-(aminomethyl)-5-methylhexanoic acid, also known as (S)-3-isobutyl GABA], is structurally related to gabapentin. It was introduced into clinical practice in 2004 for the treatment of certain types of peripheral neuropathic pain, generalised anxiety disorders and as an adjunctive therapy for focal seizures with or without secondarily generalisation.

Authorised indications

EMEA-SmPC: adjunctive therapy in adults with focal seizures with or without secondary generalisation.
FDA-PI: adjunctive therapy in adults with focal-onset seizures.

Clinical applications[229–232]

Post-marketing experience is still very limited and it appears that pregabalin is a narrow-spectrum AED that exaggerates myoclonus. Therefore, pregabalin should be only used in rational polytherapy in adults with intractable focal seizures who have failed to respond to other preferred AED combinations.

> *Treatment-emergent myoclonic jerks, even in patients with focal seizures,[233,234] may be a warning sign against the use of pregabalin in generalised and other myoclonic epilepsies, where myoclonus is often a prominent symptom to treat.*

Dosage and titration

Adults: start treatment with 150 mg/day and, based on individual patient response and tolerability, increase to 300 mg/day after an interval of 7 days, and to a maximum dose of 600 mg/day after an additional 7-day interval. The maintenance dose is 150–600 mg/day in either two or three divided doses taken orally.

Dosage adjustments are necessary in patients with renal impairment and the elderly.

TDM: probably not needed (see page 37).
Reference range: not determined.

Main ADRs

Significant weight gain was noted in 5.6% of pregabalin-treated patients in all trials.

The most commonly reported (>10%) ADRs in placebo-controlled, double-blind studies were somnolence and dizziness. Other commonly reported (>1% and <10%) ADRs were increased appetite, euphoric mood, confusion, decreased libido, irritability, ataxia, attention disturbance, abnormal coordination, memory impairment, tremor, dysarthria, paraesthesiae, blurred vision, diplopia, vertigo, dry mouth, constipation, vomiting, flatulence, erectile dysfunction, fatigue peripheral oedema, feeling drunk and abnormal gait.

There have been reports in the postmarketing experience of hypersensitivity reactions, including cases of angioedema and Stevens–Johnson syndrome.

Hypoglycaemic medication may need to be adjusted in diabetic patients who gain weight.

> *FDA warning: All patients who are currently taking or starting on pregabalin for any indication should be monitored for notable changes in behaviour that could indicate the emergence or worsening of suicidal thoughts or behaviour or depression.*

Considerations in women

Pregnancy: category C.
Others: weight gain, which is often significant, may be associated with polycystic ovary syndrome.

Main mechanisms of action

The precise mechanism of action of pregabalin is still unclear.[235] Despite being an analogue of GABA, pregabalin is inactive at $GABA_A$ and $GABA_B$ receptors and it has no effect on GABA uptake or degradation. Pregabalin probably decreases central neuronal excitability by binding to an auxiliary subunit ($\alpha_2\delta$ protein) of a high-voltage-gated calcium channel on neurones in the CNS. It reduces the release of certain neurotransmitters including glutamate, noradrenaline and substance P.

Pharmacokinetics

Oral bioavailability: >90%.
Protein binding: does not bind to plasma proteins.
Metabolism: pregabalin is not metabolised in the liver and does not induce hepatic enzymes. It is excreted renally.
Elimination half-life: 6 or 7 hours.

Drug interactions

Pregabalin does not affect the plasma concentration of other AEDs.[236] In addition, it does not interact with a number of other drug types, including hormonal contraception.

However, pregabalin appears to have an additive effect on the impairment of cognitive and gross motor function when co-administered with oxycodone (an opioid), and it potentiates the effect of lorazepam and ethanol.

Patients with galactose intolerance, glucose–galactose malabsorption or Lapp lactase deficiency should not take pregabalin.

Main disadvantages

It is still early to make any predictions for the role of pregabalin in the treatment of focal epilepsies. However, the high incidence of weight gain (consider the decline in the use of valproate because of this side effect and its causative relation with polycystic ovary syndrome in women), treatment-emergent myoclonic jerks and similarities with gabapentin[237] are not promising signs.

Rufinamide

17

Rufinamide[238–242] is a triazole derivative structurally unrelated to any currently marketed AED.

Authorised indications

EMEA-SmPC/FDA-PI: adjunctive treatment of seizures associated with Lennox–Gastaut syndrome in patients 4 years and older.

Clinical applications

Rufinamide is one of the latest AEDs marketed for the treatment of epileptic seizures. Its licenced indications are for Lennox–Gastaut syndrome, but the next step will probably be for adjunctive treatment of intractable focal epilepsies.

Dosage and titration

A lower maximum dose of rufinamide is recommended for patients being co-administered valproate, which significantly decreases clearance of rufinamide, particularly in patients with a low body weight of <30 kg.

Adults and children >30 kg: start treatment with a daily dose of 400 mg, which may be increased by increments of 400 mg/day as frequently as every 2 days, to up to a maximum recommended dose of 1800 mg/day (in the 30–50 kg weight range), 2400 mg/day (50.1–70 kg) or 3200 (>70 kg).

Children <30 kg not receiving valproate: start with a daily dose of 200 mg, which may be increased by increments of 200 mg/day as frequently as every 2 days, up to a maximum recommended dose of 1000 mg/day.

Children <30 kg also receiving valproate: start with a daily dose of 200 mg, which after a minimum of 2 days may be increased by 200 mg/day, to the maximum recommended dose of 400 mg/day.

Dosing: twice daily. Tablets can be crushed and administered in half a glass of water.

TDM: unknown.

Reference range: unknown.

Main ADRs

Frequent and/or important: headache, dizziness, fatigue, somnolence, ataxia and gait disturbances.

Serious: status epilepticus has been observed during clinical development studies, which led to the discontinuation of rufinamide in 20% of cases and none in the placebo group.

Idiosyncratic reactions and hypersensitivity syndrome (rash and fever with other organ system involvement; e.g. lymphadenopathy, liver function test abnormalities and haematuria may rarely occur with rufinamide).

Rufinamide is contraindicated in patients with familial short QT syndrome. Formal cardiac ECG studies demonstrated shortening of the QT interval (by up to 20 msec) with rufinamide treatment. Reductions of the QT interval below 300 msec were not observed in the formal QT studies with doses up to 7200 mg/day. Moreover, there was no signal for drug-induced sudden death or ventricular arrhythmias.

Considerations in women

Pregnancy: category C.
Breastfeeding: unknown but it is likely to be excreted in the breast milk.
Interactions with hormonal contraception: yes.

Mechanism of action

Rufinamide reduces the recovery capacity of neuronal sodium channels after inactivation, prolonging their inactive state by limiting neuronal sodium-dependent action potential firing.

Pharmacokinetics

Oral bioavailability: is dose dependent; as the dose increases, the bioavailability decreases. Food increases the bioavailability of rufinamide by approximately 34% and the peak plasma concentration by 56%.
Protein binding: 34%.
Metabolism: rufinamide is extensively metabolised but has no active metabolites. The primary biotransformation pathway is carboxylesterase(s)-mediated hydrolysis of the carboxylamide group to the acid derivative CGP 47292. There is no involvement of oxidizing cytochrome P450 enzymes or glutathione in the biotransformation process.

Rufinamide is a weak inhibitor of CYP 2E1. It did not show significant inhibition of other CYP enzymes. Rufinamide is a weak inducer of CYP 3A4 enzymes.
Excretion: predominantly renal (85% of the dose).
Elimination half-life: 6–10 hours.

Drug interactions

Rufinamide does not have clinically relevant effects on other AEDs but may decrease phenytoin clearance and increase average steady-state plasma concentrations of co-administered phenytoin.

However, other AEDs significantly affect rufinamide plasma concentrations, which are decreased by co-administration with carbamazepine, phenobarbital, primidone, phenytoin or vigabatrin.

Conversely, rufinamide plasma concentrations significantly increase with valproate co-administration and these are pronounced in patients of low body weight (<30 kg).

No significant changes in the concentration of rufinamide are observed following co-administration with lamotrigine, topiramate or benzodiazepines.

Patients treated with drugs that are metabolised by the CYP3A enzyme system should be carefully monitored for 2 weeks at the start of, or after the end of, treatment with rufinamide or after any marked change in the dose. A dose adjustment of the concomitantly administered drug may need to be considered. These recommendations should also be considered when rufinamide is used concomitantly with drugs with a narrow therapeutic window, such as warfarin and digoxin. No data on the interaction of rufinamide with alcohol are available.

Rufinamide interferes with hormonal contraception. Women on hormonal contraceptives are advised to use an additional safe and effective contraceptive method.

Main disadvantages

Development of status epilepticus, idiosyncratic reactions that may be serious and significant interactions with enzyme inducers (they reduce its plasma concentration) and valproate (it increases its plasma concentration).

Stiripentol[243-248]

4,4-Dimethyl-1-[3,4-(methylenedioxy)-phenyl]-1-penten-3-ol was selected for possible antiepileptic effects from a series of alpha-ethylene alcohols. Stiripentol has been known for over 30 years but because of significant problems, it was only licensed in 2009 in Europe as an adjunct-AED for Dravet syndrome, under the brand name Diacomit.

Authorised indications

SmPC: use in conjunction with clobazam and valproate as adjunctive therapy for refractory generalised tonic-clonic seizures in patients with severe myoclonic epilepsy in infancy (Dravet syndrome) whose seizures are not adequately controlled with clobazam and valproate.
FDA: Not yet approved.

Clinical applications

Limited to GTCS of Dravet syndrome. There are no clinical study data to support it as monotherapy in Dravet syndrome or other epilepsies. Studies in adult patients are disappointing.

Dosage and titration

Patients aged 3–18 years: Start with 10–20 mg/kg/day in 2–3 divided doses and increase over 3 days using upwards dose escalation to reach the recommended dose of 50 mg/kg/day administered in 2 or 3 divided doses in conjunction with clobazam and valproate.

There are no clinical study data to support its safety at doses greater than 50mg/kg/day.
Dosing: two or three times daily.
TDM: unknown.
Reference range: unknown.

Main ADRs

Frequent and/or important: anorexia, weight loss, insomnia, drowsiness, ataxia, hypotonia, dystonia and vomiting.
Serious: rash, potentiation of serious ADRs of valproate in young age groups. Transient aplastic anaemia and leukopenia have also been reported.

Considerations in women

Probably not relevant for this drug as it is licensed for Dravet syndrome only.

C.P. Panayiotopoulos, *Antiepileptic Drugs, Pharmacopoeia*,
© Springer-Verlag London Limited 2011

Pregnancy: category C.
Breastfeeding: unknown but possibly excreted in breast milk (animal data).
Interactions with hormonal contraception: yes.

Main mechanisms of action

Not fully elucidated. Direct antiepileptic effect is attributed to increase GABA levels in the brain through inhibition of synaptosomal uptake of GABA and/or inhibition of GABA transaminase. Its indirect efficacy in polytherapy is through increasing levels of other AEDs.

Pharmacokinetics

Oral bioavailability: easily and quickly absorbed but absolute bioavailability is unknown.
Protein binding: 99%
Metabolism: extensively metabolised mainly through demethylenation and glucuronidation (see below for drug interactions). Most is excreted in the urine.
Elimination half-life: 4.5 hours to 13 hours, increasing with dose.

Drug interactions

Multiple, complex and of high clinical significance. Stiripentol inhibits several cytochrome P450 isoenzymes such as CYP2C19, CYP2D6 and CYP3A4 and thus interacts with many AEDs (phenobarbital, phenytoin, carbamazepine, diazepines, tiagabine, valproate) and other medicines (theophyline, antihistamines such as astemizole, chlorpheniramine and many others), increasing their plasma levels with potential risk of overdose. It inhibits the metabolism of clobazam and its N-desmethylclobazam biotransformation, thus increasing their plasma concentrations.

Main disadvantage

Extremely difficult to use because of numerous drug interactions and of doubtful efficacy other than for its limited licensed indication.

Sulthiame

19

The story of sulthiame's transition from a disgraced to a useful drug is interesting.[249–253]

Sulthiame is a sulfonamide derivative with carbonic anhydrase-inhibiting properties (it is only one-sixteenth as potent as acetazolamide). It was first introduced as an AED in the 1960s, but its use was largely abandoned in the 1970s on the assumption that it had little, if any, anti-epileptic activity when used alone. Its anti-epileptic action was attributed to raised levels of concomitant medication (phenytoin, phenobarbital and primidone).[254,255] The significant improvement in the disturbed behaviour of mentally handicapped patients was debated and attributed to the sedative effect of sulthiame.[254] Reports that sulthiame, even in monotherapy, was a very effective drug in intractable epilepsies of infancy and childhood[256] were ignored.

Recently, sulthiame appears to have experienced a revitalisation with reports (including class 1 evidence) that it is probably the most effective drug in benign childhood focal epilepsies with regard to its effect in suppressing seizures and EEG abnormalities.[250–253] Sulthiame has also re-emerged as an AED in adults.[249]

Authorised indications

It is licensed in Australia, Germany, Ireland, Israel, and some other countries, but not by the EMEA or FDA or in the UK.

Clinical applications

Mainly in benign childhood focal epilepsies,[250–252] and epileptic encephalopathies, particularly those with EEG continuous spike–wave during sleep.[253] It may also be useful in some myoclonic epilepsies.[256]

Dosage and titration

Adults: start treatment with 250 mg and increase to 750–1000 mg. The recommended doses are much lower today than they were in the 1970s (200–600 mg/day compared to 600–3600 mg/day).

Children: 10–20 mg/day (this may also be high; a daily dose of 5 mg/kg is usually very efficacious and safe in children).

Dosing: two or three times daily.

TDM: not needed.

Reference range: it has not been precisely determined but may be around 4.1 mg/l (2.2–6.1 mg/l).

Clearance of sulthiame in children is higher than in adults and thus a higher dose/kg of sulthiame is needed to obtain an effective plasma concentration.

Main ADRs

Frequent and/or important: unsteadiness and giddiness, numbness, nausea, paraesthesiae of the face and limbs, hyperventilation (rapid or deep breathing), loss of appetite and weight loss, and rash.

Serious: idiosyncratic reactions as with other sulfonamides; metabolic acidosis and nephrolithiasis as with other carbonic anhydrase inhibitors.

Considerations in women

Pregnancy: category D.

Mechanism of action

The main mechanism of the anti-epileptic effect of sulthiame is unclear and may be multiple. Sulthiame inhibits the enzyme carbonic anhydrase in glial cells, increases the carbon dioxide concentration and leads to an acidification of the extracellular fluid. This results in a reduction of the inward currents operated by NMDA receptors and calcium currents, causing a depression of intrinsic neuronal excitability. Sulthiame has also been found to inhibit voltage-gated sodium channels, reduce the concentration of the excitatory neurotransmitter glutamate in the hippocampus of rats and guinea pigs, as well as the concentration of GABA in cerebral hemispheres of mice.

Pharmacokinetics

Oral bioavailability: 100%.
Protein binding: 29%.
Metabolism: hepatic.
Excretion: renal.
Elimination half-life: 5–10 hours (in children younger than 12 years) and 9–15 hours (in patients older than 12 years).

Drug interactions

These are significant. Sulthiame inhibits the metabolism of phenytoin, phenobarbital and primidone, so these drugs are elevated to 'therapeutic' or 'toxic' levels, or rise steeply when sulthiame is introduced.[255]

Main disadvantages

Serious drug–drug interactions and lack of licensed indications by the FDA and EMEA.

Tiagabine

20

Tiagabine [(R)-*N*-(4,4-di-(3-methyl-thien-2-yl)-but-3-enyl)nipecotic acid hydrochloride] was first licensed as an AED in 1998.[257]

Authorised indications
EMEA-SmPC/FDA-PI: adjunctive therapy for focal seizures in patients >12 years of age.

Clinical applications
The anti-epileptic efficacy of tiagabine is limited to focal seizures. Its role in clinical epileptology is probably limited to adjunctive medication in severe forms of focal epilepsies that failed to respond to other AED combinations.[258,259] It may also be effective in epileptic spasms of epileptic encephalopathies.

Dosage and titration
Dosage and titration depend on co-medication.
Adults: start treatment with 4–5 mg/day for the first week. Titrate in increments of 4–5 mg/day every week in two divided doses up to a total of 30–45 mg/day (in co-medication with enzyme-inducing drugs) or 15–30 mg/day (with non-enzyme-inducing drugs).
Children: start treatment with 0.1 mg/kg/day and titrate in increments of 0.1 mg/kg/day every 1 or 2 weeks up to a total of 0.5–2 mg/kg/day.
   Children eliminate tiagabine more rapidly than adults.
Dosing: twice or preferably three and sometimes four times daily.
TDM: not useful.
Reference range: 80–450 µg/l (50–250 nmol/l).

Main ADRs
Frequent and/or important: fatigue, headache, dizziness, tremor, cognitive impairment, disturbed concentration, depression and word-finding difficulties.
Serious: none. Concerns that tiagabine, like vigabatrin (another GABAergic AED), may cause visual field defects have not been substantiated.[260,261]
Seizure exacerbation: treatment-emergent absence status epilepticus has been reported in a significant number of patients. An opinion by a panel of experts that 'treatment with tiagabine in recommended doses does not increase the risk of status epilepticus in patients with partial seizures'[262] probably refers to focal status epilepticus and not to generalised absence status epilepticus, where the main risk lies.[263,264]

All patients who are currently taking or starting on tiagabine for any indication should be monitored for notable changes in behaviour that could indicate the emergence or worsening of suicidal thoughts or behaviour or depression.

Considerations in women

Pregnancy: category C.
Interaction with hormonal contraception: no.

Main mechanisms of action

Tiagabine is an AED specifically designed to increase GABA longevity in the synaptic cleft. It is a potent and selective inhibitor of GABA uptake into neurones and glial cells. This brain GABAergic-mediated inhibition of tiagabine explains its anti-epileptic effect on focal seizures and also explains its pro-absence effect (see useful note on page 6).[263,264]

Pharmacokinetics

Oral bioavailability: <96%. High fat meals slow the rate of absorption.
Protein binding: 96%. Salicylic acid and naprofen displace tiagabine.
Metabolism: tiagabine is metabolised by hepatic CYP before conjugation to inactive metabolites excreted in the urine and faeces. It is neither an hepatic enzyme inducer nor an inhibitor.
Elimination half-life: 7–9 hours, which decreases to 2 or 3 hours in the presence of hepatic enzyme inducers. The metabolism of tiagabine is reduced in patients with hepatic dysfunction, thus prolonging its half-life to 12–16 hours.

Drug interactions

Enzyme-inducing AEDs (phenytoin, carbamazepine and phenobarbital) significantly lower the plasma concentrations of tiagabine by a factor of 1.5–3 and shorten its half-life.

Valproate displaces tiagabine from its protein-binding sites.

Tiagabine does not affect other AEDs or hormonal contraception.

Main disadvantages

- Narrow-spectrum anti-epileptic efficacy against focal seizures only. Its use is prohibiited in IGE with absences because tiagabine is a pro-absence drug.
- Multiple drug interactions and complicated dosage and titration schemes.

Topiramate

21

Topiramate is a sulfamate-substituted monosaccharide designated chemically as 2,3:4,5-di-*O*-isopropylidene-β-D-fructopyranose sulfamate. It was first introduced into clinical practice in 1995.

Authorised indications

UK-SmPC: (1) monotherapy in patients ≥6 years of age with newly diagnosed epilepsy who have GTCSs or focal seizures with or without secondarily generalised seizures; (2) adjunctive therapy in patients ≥2 years of age who are inadequately controlled on conventional first-line AEDs for focal seizures with or without secondarily generalised seizures, seizures associated with Lennox–Gastaut syndrome and primary GTCSs. The efficacy and safety of conversion from adjunctive therapy to topiramate monotherapy has not been demonstrated.

FDA-PI: (1) initial monotherapy for focal onset or primary GTCSs in patients ≥10 of age; effectiveness was demonstrated in a controlled trial in patients with epilepsy who had no more than 2 seizures in the 3 months prior to enrollment. Safety and effectiveness in patients who were converted to monotherapy from a previous regimen of other anticonvulsant drugs have not been established in controlled trials; (2) adjunctive therapy for adults and pediatric patients ages 2–16 years with partial onset seizures, or primary generalised tonic–clonic seizures, and in patients 2 years of age and older with seizures associated with Lennox–Gastaut syndrome.

Clinical applications

Topiramate is a highly efficacious new, broad-spectrum AED, but significant ADRs hinder its clinical use.[265–273] It is probably the most effective of all the newer AEDs in focal seizures. In clinical use, topiramate has been recommended for all types of seizures – focal or generalised, and idiopathic or symptomatic – in adults and children including difficult-to-treat epileptic encephalopathies, such as West and Lennox–Gastaut syndromes.

Dosage and titration

'Start very low and go very slow' is particularly important. Treatment with topiramate should be initiated at a very low dosage and be titrated at a very slow pace. If the patient is unable to tolerate the titration regimen, smaller increments or longer intervals between increments can be used. Maintenance doses are usually reached in 2 months.

Adults and children over 16 years: start with 25 mg nocte for the first week and then titrate in increments of 25 or 50 mg/day in two equally divided doses at 1 or 2 week intervals. The recommended maintenance dose is 200–400 mg/day. Some authors recommend a maximum dose of 800 mg/day, but this is rarely tolerated. *Children 6–16 years:* start treatment with 25 mg or 1–3 mg/kg/day nocte for the first week. Titrate with increments of 1–3 mg/kg/day in two divided doses at 1- or 2-week intervals to a recommended maintenance dose of 5–9 mg/kg/day in two divided doses. *Children 2–6 years:* start with 0.5–1 mg/kg/day nocte for the first week and then titrate as for older children. *Renally impaired patients:* half of the usual dose is recommended. Patients with moderate or severe renal impairment may take 10–15 days to reach steady-state plasma concentrations compared with 4–8 days in patients with normal renal function.

Tablets should not be broken.

Therapy should not be withdrawn suddenly because of the risk of aggravating seizures.

Dosing: twice daily.

TDM: probably not needed (see page 37).

Reference range: 9–12 mg/l (15–60 µmol/l).

Main ADRs

Topiramate is an inferior newer AED with respect to ADRs, which are common, multiple and sometimes severe or potentially fatal.[274,275] Withdrawal rates were low in controlled trials (4.8%),[266,276] but appear to be much more frequent in non-comparative and post-marketing studies.[265,277] On the positive side, topiramate lacks significant idiosyncratic reactions.

Frequent and/or important: somnolence, anorexia, fatigue and nervousness are common as in other AEDs, but most of the other frequent ADRs are of concern.

Serious: ADRs are numerous and diverse.

Abnormal thinking, consisting of mental slowing and word-finding difficulties, has been reported in 31% of patients with titration rates of 100 mg per week.[278,279]

Difficulty with concentration/attention, memory impairment, psychomotor slowing and speech disorders are often very severe, even when treatment starts with small doses and titration is slow.

Behavioural and cognitive problems are a limiting factor in some children. Topiramate was reported to have a negative impact on cognition with impairment of performance on tests requiring verbal processing, which was consistent with subjective complaints of patients.[280–281]

Weight loss (10% of patients) may be considered as beneficial by some women, but is sometimes relentless and extremely problematic.[265] A dietary supplement or increased food intake may be considered if the patient is losing weight or has inadequate weight gain while receiving topiramate.

Treatment-emergent paraesthesiae and abdominal pains may be confused with other systemic disorders.

Metabolic acidosis: hyperchloraemic, non-anion gap, metabolic acidosis (i.e. decreased serum bicarbonate below the normal reference range in the absence of respiratory alkalosis) is associated with use of topiramate. The incidence of persistent treatment-emergent decreases in serum bicarbonate is high and rises significantly with increasing topiramate dosages. Generally, the decrease in bicarbonate occurs early in treatment, although it can occur at any time during treatment.

Markedly abnormal low serum bicarbonate levels (i.e. an absolute value of <17 mEq/l and >5 mEq/l decrease from pretreatment levels) occurred in 11% of children receiving topiramate 6 mg/kg/day and 3% of adults receiving 400 mg/ day. In placebo-controlled trials of migraine prophylaxis in adults, markedly abnormally low serum bicarbonate levels occurred in 11% of those receiving 200 mg/day, 9% on 100 mg/day, 2% on 50 mg/day and <1% with placebo.

Diseases or therapies that predispose to acidosis, such as renal disease, severe respiratory disorders, status epilepticus, diarrhoea, surgery, ketogenic diet or certain drugs (e.g. zonisamide) may be additive to the bicarbonate-lowering effects of topiramate.

Manifestations of acute or chronic metabolic acidosis may include hyperventilation, non-specific symptoms, such as fatigue and anorexia, or more severe sequelae including cardiac arrhythmias or stupor.

Depending on the underlying conditions, appropriate evaluation, including serum bicarbonate levels is recommended with topiramate therapy.

> *Chronic, untreated metabolic acidosis may increase the risk of nephrolithiasis or nephrocalcinosis, and may also result in osteomalacia (rickets in paediatric patients) and/or osteoporosis with an increased risk of fractures. Chronic metabolic acidosis in paediatric patients may also reduce growth rates.*
> *A reduction in growth rate may eventually decrease the maximal height achieved. The effect of topiramate on growth and bone-related sequelae is unknown and has not been systematically investigated.*

Nephrolithiasis: around 1.5% of adults and 0.6% children in clinical trials of topiramate developed renal stones. Risk factors for nephrolithiasis include prior stone formation, a family history of nephrolithiasis and hypercalciuria. None of these risk factors can reliably predict stone formation during topiramate treatment. In addition, patients taking other medication associated with nephrolithiasis, such as zonisamide, may be at increased risk.

Topiramate, like other carbonic anhydrase inhibitors, reduces urinary citrate excretion and increases urinary pH.

> *Patients receiving topiramate should increase their fluid intake because this may reduce the risk of: (1) developing renal stones; and (2) heat-related adverse events during exercise and exposure to particularly warm environments.*

Acute myopia with secondary angle-closure glaucoma is a syndrome reported in adults and children treated with topiramate.[282] Symptoms typically occur within 1 month of the start of treatment and include acute onset of decreased visual acuity and/or ocular pain. Ophthalmological findings include bilateral myopia, anterior chamber shallowing, ocular hyperaemia and increased intra-ocular pressure with or without mydriasis. There may be supraciliary effusion resulting in anterior displacement of the lens and iris. Discontinuation of topiramate should be as rapid as is clinically feasible. Immediate specialist advice should be sought. If left untreated, elevated intra-ocular pressure can lead to serious sequelae, including permanent visual loss.

Oligohidrosis and hyperthermia: hypohidrosis or, more seriously, anhidrosis associated with hyperthermia, which infrequently results in hospitalisation, has been reported in association with topiramate. Symptoms include decreased or absence of sweating, elevation of body temperature, red face and tiredness, which worsen with exertion.

The majority of the reports have been in children and have occurred after exposure to hot environmental conditions. Patients, especially children, treated with topiramate should be monitored closely for evidence of such symptoms especially in hot weather.

Caution should be used when topiramate is prescribed with other drugs that predispose patients to heat-related disorders, such as zonisamide (such a combination should probably be avoided), other carbonic anhydrase inhibitors and anticholinergic drugs.

> *FDA warning: All patients who are currently taking or starting on topiramate for any indication should be monitored for notable changes in behaviour that could indicate the emergence or worsening of suicidal thoughts or behaviour or depression.*

Considerations in women

Pregnancy: category C. There is no reliable information on human teratogenicity, but in animals even subtoxic doses of topiramate are teratogenic.[283]

Breastfeeding: breastfeeding is not recommended because of extensive secretion of topiramate into breast milk.

Interactions with hormonal contraception: there is a dose-dependent decrease in ethinyl estradiol exposure with topiramate doses between 200 and 800 mg/day, which may result in decreased efficacy of hormonal contraception or increased breakthrough bleeding.

Main mechanisms of action

The anti-epileptic effect of topiramate is probably due to multimodal mechanisms of action. These include blockage of voltage-dependent sodium channels, augmentation of the inhibitory activity of GABA at some subtypes of the GABA$_A$

receptor, antagonism with the AMPA/kainate subtype of the glutamate receptor, and inhibition of the carbonic anhydrase enzyme, particularly isozymes II and IV.

Pharmacokinetics

Oral bioavailability: >80%.

Protein binding: 15–41% over the blood concentration range of 0.5–250 µg/ml. The fraction bound decreases as blood concentration increases.

Metabolism: topiramate is not extensively metabolised and is primarily eliminated unchanged in the urine (approximately 70% of an administered dose). Six metabolites have been identified in humans, none of which constitutes more than 5% of an administered dose. The metabolites are formed via hydroxylation, hydrolysis and glucuronidation. There is evidence of renal tubular reabsorption of topiramate.

Elimination half-life: 21 hours.

Drug interactions

The following anti-epileptic drug–drug interactions are of clinical significance with topiramate co-medication:

- In co-medication, phenytoin plasma levels may increase by 25% and topiramate decrease by 48%. Carbamazepine may decrease topiramate plasma by nearly a half.
- There is probably no interaction with lamotrigine and levetiracetam, and interactions with valproate are minimal.
- Concomitant use with other carbonic anhydrase inhibitors, such as zonisamide, should probably be avoided.

Main disadvantages

Despite high efficacy, the current and future role of topiramate as a major AED is questionable, because of its very-poor profile in terms of multiple and severe ADRs. The most important of these reactions are those that occur in children, some of which (metabolic acidosis) may have predictable detrimental growth and bone-related sequelae in long-term use.

Its use may be limited to severe epilepsies intractable to other, better tolerated, AEDs.

Valproate

The introduction of valproate as an AED in the early 1960s revolutionised the treatment of generalised epilepsies.[284–285] Valproic acid (2-propyl pentanoic acid, 2-propyl valeric acid) is a short-chain branched fatty acid. Prior to the serendipitous discovery of its anti-epileptic activity in 1963, valproic acid was used as an organic solvent.

Valproate is a general term used to include all available forms of valproic acid, such as sodium valproate, magnesium valproate and sodium divalproex.

Authorised indications

UK-SmPC: In the treatment of generalised, partial or other epilepsy.
FDA-PI: (1) monotherapy and adjunctive therapy in the treatment of patients with complex partial seizures that occur either in isolation or in association with other types of seizures and (2) use as sole and adjunctive therapy in the treatment of simple and complex absence seizures, and adjunctively in patients with multiple seizure types which include absence seizures.

Simple absence is defined as very brief clouding of the sensorium or loss of consciousness accompanied by certain generalised epileptic discharges without other detectable clinical signs. Complex absence is the term used when other signs are also present.

Valproate sodium injection is indicated as an intravenous alternative in patients for whom oral administration of valproate products is temporarily not feasible.

Clinical applications

Valproate is one of the most effective broad-spectrum AEDs for all types of seizures and epilepsies. It has superior efficacy in all types of generalised seizures (idiopathic and symptomatic), all syndromes of IGE and photosensitive epilepsy compared with any other drug so far, with the probable exception of levetiracetam. The efficacy of valproate has been well documented in long-term and worldwide clinical practice and controlled studies.

However, valproate is (1) far inferior to carbamazepine and some newer AEDs in the treatment of focal epilepsies and (2) has serious ADRs in women of child-bearing age and in patients of early childhood.

Unlike many other AEDs, valproate appears to have a very low potential to aggravate seizures.[287] When seizure aggravation occurs with valproate, it is in a specific clinical context, such as overdose, encephalopathy, or hepatic or metabolic disorders.[287]

C.P. Panayiotopoulos, *Antiepileptic Drugs, Pharmacopoeia,*
© Springer-Verlag London Limited 2011

Dosage and titration

Adults: start treatment with 200 mg/day in two equally divided doses for 3 days. Titrate in increments of 200 mg/day every 3 days to a maintenance dose of usually 1000–1500 mg/day (maximum 3000 mg/day) given in two equally divided doses. Higher initial dosage and faster titration rates are usually well tolerated.

Children: start with 10 mg/kg/day. Titrate in increments of 10 mg/kg/day every 3 days. The typical maintenance dose in childhood is 20–30 mg/kg/day in two equally divided doses.

Combined therapy: it may be necessary to increase the dose by 30–50% when used in combination with enzyme-inducing AEDs, such as phenytoin, phenobarbital and carbamazepine. On withdrawal of these AEDs, it may be possible to reduce the dose of valproate.

Dosing: twice or three times daily, and once daily for slow-release formulations.

TDM: often not useful, because of poor correlation between valproate dose and plasma levels. However, because of significant drug interactions, monitoring of valproate and AEDs given concomitantly may be helpful when enzyme-inducing drugs are added or withdrawn.

Reference range (measures valproic acid): 50–100 mg/l (300–700 μmol/l).

Main ADRs

> *Valproate is associated with serious ADRs, particularly in children and women. Acute liver necrosis and acute pancreatitis, which may be fatal, are rare and more likely to occur in children receiving polypharmacy. An estimated 1–2% risk of neural tube defects, predominantly spina bifida aperta, in babies of women on valproate is well established,[288,289] and the overall risk of major teratogenic effects with valproate is two to three times higher than the background prevalence of major non-syndromic congenital anomalies.[16] This, together with polycystic ovary syndrome, and other endocrine ADRs,[291] makes the use of valproate in some women undesirable.*

CNS-related ADRs: in contrast with other older AEDs, valproate is not usually associated with drowsiness and fatigability or significant dose-related effects on cognition or behaviour. Valproate encephalopathy is exceptional.

Tremor is the more troublesome CNS adverse effect of valproate. There is great individual susceptibility to the development of tremor, which is usually mild, but may become very intense, socially embarrassing and disabling. It is reversible and declines when the dose is lowered.

Systemic: the most serious are fatal hepatotoxicity and acute haemorrhagic pancreatitis.

Hepatic failure resulting in fatalities is primarily age-dependent and occurs mainly in children receiving polypharmacy and with organic brain disease. The risk is 1/600 before the age of 3 years. The incidence of fatal hepatotoxicity decreases considerably in progressively older patient groups (range 1/8000–1/10,000 between 3 and 20 years of age) and in monotherapy with valproate.

Hepatic failure has usually occurred during the first 6 months of treatment. The diagnosis is based on clinical criteria with non-specific symptoms, such as malaise, weakness, lethargy, facial oedema, anorexia, vomiting and loss of seizure control. Liver function tests should be performed prior to therapy and at frequent intervals thereafter, especially during the first 6 months. However, this may not be helpful because:

- benign elevation of liver enzymes is common during valproate treatment
- severe hepatotoxicity is not preceded by progressive elevation of liver enzymes.

Raised liver enzymes are common during treatment with valproate, particularly if used in conjunction with other AEDs. These are usually transient or respond to dose reduction. Patients with such biochemical abnormalities should be reassessed clinically and liver function tests should be performed more frequently. An abnormally low prothrombin level, particularly in association with other relevant abnormalities, requires withdrawal of valproate. Any concomitant use of salicylates should be stopped, since they employ the same metabolic pathway.

Acute haemorrhagic pancreatitis with markedly increased amylase and lipase levels is another rare, but serious, adverse effect of valproate treatment. It develops within the first 3 months of treatment, is more prevalent in children and with polytherapy.

Hyperammonaemic encephalopathy, which is sometimes fatal, has been reported following initiation of valproate therapy in patients with urea cycle disorders. When urea cycle enzymatic deficiency is suspected, metabolic investigations should be performed prior to treatment with valproate.

Thrombocytopenia and other haematological abnormalities:[292] it is recommended that platelet counts and coagulation tests are performed before initiating therapy and at periodic intervals, because of reports of thrombocytopenia, inhibition of the secondary phase of platelet aggregation and abnormal coagulation parameters. Evidence of haemorrhage, bruising or a disorder of haemostasis/ coagulation is an indication for reduction or withdrawal of valproate.

Weight gain occurs in 20% of patients and is sometimes marked; women are more vulnerable. This is usually reversible if valproate is withdrawn early.

Hair loss and changes in hair texture or colour are relatively rare; they usually occur in the early months of valproate treatment and may resolve spontaneously despite continuation of the drug.

Other ADRs concern the gastrointestinal system (e.g. anorexia, constipation, dry mouth, stomatitis) and urogenital system (e.g. urinary incontinence, vaginitis, dysmenorrhoea, amenorrhoea and urinary frequency).

FDA warning: All patients who are currently taking or starting on valproate for any indication should be monitored for notable changes in behaviour that could indicate the emergence or worsening of suicidal thoughts or behaviour or depression.

Considerations in women

Valproate treatment in women raises many issues, as has been detailed on many occassions in the literature and in the booklet, *Principles of Therapy in the Epilepsies.*

Pregnancy: category D.[288,289,293] Valproate is teratogenic. It crosses the placenta and causes a spectrum of congenital anomalies, such as neural tube defects, craniofacial malformations and skeletal defects. The incidence of these anomalies is much higher when valproate is given as co-medication with other AEDs.

Breastfeeding: There appears to be no contra-indication to breast feeding; excretion in breast milk is low and with no clinical effects.

Interaction with hormonal contraception: none.

Other issues: see endocrine abnormalities.

Main mechanisms of action

The main mechanism of action is unknown and a combination of several mechanisms may be responsible:

- reduction of sustained, repetitive, high-frequency firing by inhibiting voltage-sensitive sodium channels, activating calcium-dependent potassium conductance and possibly by direct action on other ion channels
- valproate has a GABAergic effect through elevation of brain GABA by various mechanisms, such as inhibiting GABA-transaminase (GABA-T), enhancing GABA-synthesising enzymes, increasing GABA release and inhibiting GABA uptake. However, this GABAergic action is observed only at high valproate levels and may explain its efficacy in other, but not absence, seizures. GABAergic drugs that affect $GABA_B$ receptors have a pro-absence action because they potentiate absences (see useful note on page 6). Another explanation for the effect of valproate on absence seizures is that this drug, like ethosuximide, reduces a low threshold (T-type) calcium-channel current,[294] but this effect has not been supported by other studies.[295]

Pharmacokinetics

Oral bioavailability: almost complete. Absorption of valproate varies according to the formulation used. Absorption is rapid and peak levels are reached within 2 hours after oral administration of syrup or uncoated tablets. This is longer (3–8 hours) with enteric-coated tablets.

Protein binding: valproate is highly protein bound (about 90%). However, if the plasma level of valproic acid rises above 120 mg/l or if the serum albumin concentration is lowered, the binding sites may become saturated, causing the amount of free drug to rise rapidly, out of proportion to any increase in dosage. Valproate may displace phenobarbital or phenytoin from plasma protein-binding sites.

Metabolism: hepatic. Valproate has a complex metabolism. It is rapidly and nearly totally eliminated by hepatic metabolism with numerous metabolites that contribute to its efficacy and toxicity. Two metabolites of valproate, 2-ene-valproic acid and 4-ene-valproic, are among the most pharmacologically active and have a similar potency to the parent drug. They are both produced by the action of CYP enzymes induced by other AEDs. They are eliminated primarily in the urine.

The major elimination pathway is via glucuronidation (40–60%). The remainder is largely metabolised via oxidation pathways, β-oxidation accounting for 30–40% and ϖ-oxidation, which is CYP dependent. Only 1–3% of the ingested dose is excreted unchanged in the urine.

Elimination half-life: this is variable, but generally appears to be 8–12 hours (range 4–16 hours). It is shorter in patients receiving enzyme-modifying AEDs or in long-term valproate treatment of children and adults. Many antipsychotic and antidepressant drugs result in competitive metabolism or enzyme inhibition when given as a co-medication with valproate.

Drug interactions

There are numerous drug interactions with valproate because:

- its metabolism is sensitive to enzymatic induction
- it inhibits the metabolism of other drugs
- it has a high affinity for serum proteins; it may be displaced or displace other drugs.

Effect of other AEDs on valproate: enzyme inducers, particularly those that elevate levels of UGTs, such as phenobarbital, phenytoin and carbamazepine, may increase the clearance of valproate, thus reducing plasma valproate levels by 30–50%.

The addition of ethosuximide may reduce the plasma concentration of valproate. *Effects of valproate on other AEDs:* valproate does not interact with most of the newer AEDs. A notable exception is lamotrigine.[296] Valproate is a potent inhibitor of UGT-dependent metabolism of lamotrigine, and doubles[251] or triples[76] its plasma half-life.

The addition of valproate to ethosuximide or phenobarbital may double the plasma concentration of these AEDs with concomitant toxicity.

There is evidence of severe CNS depression, with or without significant elevations of barbiturate or valproate plasma concentrations. All patients receiving concomitant barbiturate therapy should be closely monitored for neurological toxicity. Plasma barbiturate concentrations should be measured, if possible, and the barbiturate dosage decreased, if appropriate.

Plasma levels of carbamazepine decrease to around 17%, while those of carbamazepine-10,11-epoxide increase by 45% on co-administration with valproate.

Valproate displaces phenytoin from its plasma albumin-binding sites and inhibits its hepatic metabolism. Valproate significantly increases the free fraction of phenytoin and reduces its total plasma concentration.

Valproate does not interact with hormonal contraception.

Main disadvantages

The superior efficacy of valproate in generalised seizures is hindered by serious acute and chronic ADRs. It is particularly unsuitable for:

- women, because of hormonal changes, weight gain and teratogenicity; it is virtually impossible to prescribe valproate to young women today. There are increasing numbers of litigations against physicians and health authorities by parents of children with foetal valproate syndrome (even if the risks were appropriately explained to them) on a scale characterised by the media as 'bigger than thalidomide'.
- young children, particularly those <2 years, who are at a considerably increased risk of developing fatal hepatotoxicity, especially those on multiple anticonvulsants or with congenital metabolic disorders, mental retardation or organic brain disease.

Valproate is the superior AED for generalised epilepsies, but its use in focal epilepsies is of very limited value, because:

- the doses of valproate required to be effective are much higher in focal than generalised epilepsies
- ADRs, particularly in some women, make its use undesirable
- there are other, more effective and safer drugs for focal seizures.

Vigabatrin

23

Vigabatrin (γ-vilyl-GABA; 4-amino-hex-5-enoic acid) was a result of a rational approach to design compounds that enhance the effect of the inhibitory neurotransmitter GABA.[297-314]

Authorised indications
UK-SmPC: (1) monotherapy in the treatment of infantile spasms and (2) treatment in combination with other anti-epileptic drugs for patients with resistant partial epilepsy with or without secondary generalisation, where all other appropriate drug combinations have proved inadequate or have not been tolerated.
FDA-PI: not yet licensed, but expected soon.

Clinical applications
The use of vigabatrin as an AED is, in clinical practice, limited to infantile (epileptic) spasms for which it is the initial treatment of choice.[297]

Exceptionally vigabatrin may be used cautiously in the treatment of patients with intractable focal seizures that have failed to respond to all other appropriate AED combinations and surgical procedures.[297,298]

Dosage and titration
Adults: start treatment with 500 mg/day and titrate in increments of 500 mg/day every week. Typical adult maintenance dose is 1000–3000 mg/day given in two equally divided doses.

Because the excretion is mainly renal, the dose should be reduced in patients with renal insufficiency and creatinine clearance <60 ml/l.
Children with infantile spasms: start treatment with 50 mg/kg/day and adjust according to the response over 7 days, up to a total of 150–200 mg/kg/day.
Dosing: despite its short half-life (5–7 hours), vigabatrin may be given once or twice daily, because inhibition of GABA-T results in a relatively long duration of action, and GABA levels in the CSF can remain elevated for up to 120 hours after a single oral dose.
TDM: unnecessary; useful only to check compliance.[71,72]
Reference range: 6–278 μmol/l, which is irrelevant in clinical practice.

Main ADRs
Visual field defects are the main concern.[305,312] Other ADRs include sedation, dizziness, headache, ataxia, paraesthesiae, memory, cognitive and behavioural disturbances, weight gain and tremor. There is no evidence of idiosyncratic ADRs.

Visual field defects: there is a high prevalence of visual field defects occurring in around one-third of patients (adults and children)[312] treated with vigabatrin. Vigabatrin also produces retinal electrophysiological changes in nearly all patients.[260,311,312]

Visual field loss resulting from vigabatrin is not usually reversible. However, visual acuity, colour vision and the loss of amplitude on the electroretinogram may be reversible in patients with minimal or no visual field loss. There is some evidence that visual field defects remain stable with continuous treatment. It is, therefore, feasible to continue treatment with vigabatrin in these cases, provided visual field monitoring is performed regularly.[311]

In one study involving 24 children treated with vigabatrin, visual field constriction or abnormal ocular electrophysiological studies were seen in over 50% of cases.[312]

The mechanism of vigabatrin-induced visual field defects are probably due to reversible oedema of the myelin in the optic nerves, retinal cone system dysfunction or both.

Main mechanisms of action

The anti-epileptic activity of vigabatrin is by selective and irreversible inhibition of GABA-T, thus preventing the breakdown of GABA. Vigabatrin produces dose-dependent increases in GABA concentrations in the CSF and decreases in GABA-T activity. Raised brain GABA levels inhibit the propagation of abnormal hypersynchronous seizure discharges.

Vigabatrin may also cause a decrease in excitation-related amino acids.

Pharmacokinetics

Oral bioavailability: 80–100%.
Protein binding: none.
Metabolism: it is not metabolised and 70% is excreted unchanged in the urine. It is eliminated by the kidneys by glomerular filtration.
Elimination half-life: 5–8 hours (not clinically important).

Drug interactions

There are no drug interactions of any clinical significance, except for lowering the concentration of phenytoin.

Considerations in women

Pregnancy: category C.
Breastfeeding: only small amounts of the drug are excreted in breast milk.
Interactions with hormonal contraception: none.

Main disadvantages

Visual field defects have virtually eliminated vigabatrin from common clinical practice except for infantile spasms.

Aggravation of seizures: vigabatrin is a pro-absence agent which aggravates absence seizures and provokes absence status epilepticus.[310] This alone would prohibit use of vigabatrin in IGEs with absences.

Vigabatrin, in addition to its aggravation effect on typical absence seizures, may also exaggerate atypical absences (such as those occurring in Lennox–Gastaut syndrome) and myoclonic seizures (such as those occurring in progressive or non-progressive myoclonic epilepsies).

Useful clinical note

Visual field defects may not be clinically detectable. Therefore, patients should be monitored with perimetry prior to and every 6 months during vigabatrin treatment. Electrophysiological testing is considered to be more accurate than perimetry for the direct vigabatrin effect on the outer retina.[314] The manufacturers provide a procedure for testing children <9 years of age for visual field defects.

Two lessons to be learned from vigabatrin

First lesson:
Numerous RCTs failed to detect common and serious visual field defects

Vigabatrin was used as an adjunctive medication in the treatment of focal epilepsies from 1989, when it was first licensed in Europe. Concern over neuropathological findings of microvacuolisation of white matter in animals caused trials of vigabatrin to be halted in 1983, but trials were resumed when a lack of evidence (including visual-evoked responses) for toxicity in humans was found.

Numerous RCTs (mostly of class I and II in the ratings of 'therapeutic articles')[299–306] were all consistent in their conclusion that vigabatrin was a 'relatively safe drug with a relatively benign adverse-effect profile'. They all failed to identify vigabatrin-associated irreversible visual field defects. It was astute clinicians who first reported these serious ADRs,[305] but even after this report had been published, a class I RCT found vigabatrin to be 'less effective but better tolerated than carbamazepine'.[306] Results of proper testing for visual field defects are not given; that the patients did not have abnormalities on visual confrontation testing is not reassuring. When such ADRs come to light, good clinical practice mandates that patients are informed and offered the appropriate testing. Visual field testing performed by a protocol amendment post hoc (after termination of another RCT) showed abnormalities in 10% of vigabatrin-treated patients.[307]

Second lesson:
Authorities failed to warn of the pro-absence effects of vigabatrin

That vigabatrin is a pro-absence AED should be evident by its action on GABAB receptors. No such warning was given to practising physicians,[309] who only discovered this effect when patients with IGEs experienced significant deterioration and absence status epilepticus.[310]

Zonisamide

24

Zonisamide is a synthetic 1,2-benzisoxazole derivative (1,2-benzisoxazole-3-methanesulfonamide). It is chemically classified as a sulfonamide with a structural similarity to serotonin. It was first introduced as an AED in Japan in 1989.[315,316]

Efficacy, dose and mean plasma levels were similar in multi-centre studies with Japanese and Caucasian subjects.[315,317]

Authorised indications

EMEA-SmPC: Adjunctive therapy in adult patients with focal seizures with or without secondary generalisation.

FDA-PI: Adjunctive therapy in the treatment of focal seizures in adults with epilepsy.

Clinical applications[318–332]

Zonisamide appears to be an effective broad-spectrum AED with extensive clinical use in Japan. It is efficacious in focal seizures with or without GTCSs, primarily and secondarily generalised seizures including epileptic spasms of West syndrome, other epileptic encephalopathies such as Ohtahara syndrome, and probably progressive myoclonic epilepsies such as Unverricht syndrome.

Dosage and titration

'Start low and go slow' is an important part of treatment with zonisamide.[316] Significant adjustments are needed in co-medication with hepatic-enzyme inducers.

Adults: Start with 100 mg/day in one or two equally divided doses. After two weeks, the dose may be increased to 200 mg/day for at least two weeks. It can be increased to 300 mg/day and 400 mg/day, with the dose stable for at least two weeks to achieve steady state at each level. Evidence from controlled trials suggests that zonisamide doses of 100–600 mg/day are effective, but there is no suggestion of increasing response above 400 mg/day.

Because of the long half-life of zonisamide, up to two weeks may be required to achieve steady state levels upon reaching a stable dose or following dosage adjustment. Some experts prolong the duration of treatment at the lower doses in order to fully assess the effects of zonisamide at steady state, noting that many of the side effects of zonisamide are more frequent at doses of 300 mg per day and above. Although there is some evidence of greater response at doses above 100–200 mg/day, the increase appears small and formal dose-response studies have not been conducted.

Marked renal impairment (creatinine clearance <20 ml/min) requires slower dose escalation and lower maintenance doses.

Dosing: once or twice daily.

Children: start with 1–2 mg/kg/day for the first week and titrate in increments of 1–2 mg/kg/day every 2 weeks. Usual childhood maintenance dose is 4–8 mg/ kg/day (maximum 12 mg/kg/day) in two equally divided doses.

TDM: useful, although there is insufficient evidence to support a clear relation between the plasma concentration of zonisamide and clinical response.[317] Zonisamide monitoring may be needed in order to adjust the dosage in co-medication with phenytoin, phenobarbital or carbamazepine.

Reference range: 15–40 mg/l (45–180 µmol/l).

Main ADRs

Zonisamide causes many ADRs.

Frequent and/or important: sedation, somnolence, fatigue, dizziness, agitation, irritability, anorexia, weight loss, nausea, diarrhoea, dyspepsia, dry mouth, slowing of mental activity, depression, ataxia, visual hallucinations, photosensitivity, resting and postural hand tremors.

Potentially serious: some of the ADRs are similar to those of topiramate. These are:
- cognitive impairment, including word-finding difficulty; this is worse in children with plasma concentrations >140 µmol/l
- weight loss and anorexia that may become very severe
- nephrolithiasis in 4% of patients on prolonged zonisamide therapy
- oligohidrosis and anhidrosis often accompanied by hyperthermia, especially in children and hot environments.

  Additional severe ADRs are those seen with the sulfonamides, such as rash, Stevens–Johnson syndrome, toxic epidermal necrolysis and major haematological disturbances including aplastic anaemia, which very rarely can be fatal. The incidence of rash requiring discontinuation of therapy has been approximately 2% in clinical trials.

Depression and psychosis may be common, particularly in children. In one study, 14 of 74 patients experienced psychotic episodes within a few years of commencement of zonisamide.[323]

Seizure exacerbation: treatment-emergent status epilepticus has been reported in 1.1% of treated patients, compared to no reported cases in placebo-treated individuals.[298,301]

Considerations in women

Pregnancy: category C.

Breastfeeding: the transfer rate of zonisamide through breast milk is high at about 50%.

Interaction with oral hormonal contraception: none.

Main mechanisms of action

The anti-epileptic mechanism of zonisamide is probably multimodal. Zonisamide blocks the sustained repetitive firing of voltage-sensitive sodium channels and reduces voltage-dependent T-type calcium current without affecting the L-type calcium current. It has mild carbonic anhydrase activity and inhibits excitatory glutamatergic transmission. It exhibits free radical-scavenging properties.

Pharmacokinetics

Bioavailability: 100%.

Protein binding: 40–60%.

Metabolism and route of elimination: zonisamide is metabolised in the liver and eliminated by the kidneys. It is metabolised partly by CYP3A4 (reductive cleavage), and also by N-acetyl-transferases and conjugation with glucuronic acid; therefore, substances that can induce or inhibit these enzymes may affect the pharmacokinetics of zonisamide. It does not induce hepatic enzymes. Nearly half of zonisamide is excreted unchanged in the urine.

Elimination half-life: 60 hours, which decreases to 27–38 hours in the presence of hepatic enzyme inducers.

Interaction with other drugs

Plasma concentrations of zonisamide are altered by drugs that either induce or inhibit CYP3A4. Phenytoin, phenobarbital and carbamazepine increase zonisamide plasma clearance and reduce its half-life to 27–38 hours.[324] Valproate also reduces its half-life to 46 hours.

Zonisamide does not appear to affect phenytoin, but significantly increases the plasma concentration of carbamazepine epoxide when added to carbamazepine.

Concomitant administration of carbonic anhydrase inhibitors, such as acetazolamide or topiramate, is probably ill advised because of the increased potential for renal stone and metabolic acidosis.

Main disadvantages

Zonisamide has significant ADRs, some of which may be severe such as cognitive, psychotic episodes, anhidrosis and hyperthermia, nephrolithiasis and Stevens–Johnson syndrome. It also has many interactions with other AEDs in polytherapy.[324]

References

1. Shorvon S, ed. Handbook of epilepsy treatment. Second edition. Oxford: Blackwell Science, 2005.
2. Shorvon S, Perucca E, Engel JJr,eds. The treatment of epilepsy (third edition). Oxford: Wiley-Blackwell, 2009:1–1056.
3. Wyllie E, Gupta A, Lachhwani D, eds. The treatment of epilepsy. Principles and practice. Fourth edition. Philadelphia: Lippincott Williams & Wilkins, 2006.
4. Pellock JM, Bourgeois BFD, Dodson WE, eds. Pediatric epilepsy: Diagnosis and treatment (third edition). New York: Demos Medical Publishing, 2008.
5. Bialer M, Johannessen SI, Levy RH, Perucca E, Tomson T, White HS. Progress report on new antiepileptic drugs: a summary of the Ninth Eilat Conference (EILAT IX). Epilepsy Res 2009;83:1–43.
6. Panayiotopoulos CP. Treatment of typical absence seizures and related epileptic syndromes. Paediatr Drugs 2001;3:379–403.
7. Lim LL, Foldvary N, Mascha E, Lee J. Acetazolamide in women with catamenial epilepsy. Epilepsia 2001;42:746–9.
8. Shorvon S, Perucca E, Engel JJr, eds. The treatment of epilepsy (3nd edition). Oxford: Willey-Blackwell; 2009. p. 829–54.
9. Farrell K, Michoulas A. Benzodiazepines. In: Pellock JM, Bourgeois BFD, Dodson WE, editors. Pediatric epilepsy: Diagnosis and treatment. Third edition, pp 557–66. New York: Demos Medical Publishing; 2008.
10. Kaniwa N, Saito Y, Aihara M, Matsunaga K, Tohkin M et al. HLA-B locus in Japanese patients with anti-epileptics and allopurinol-related Stevens-Johnson syndrome and toxic epidermal necrolysis. Pharmacogenomics 2008;9:1617–22.
11. Ferrell PB, Jr., McLeod HL. Carbamazepine, HLA-B*1502 and risk of Stevens-Johnson syndrome and toxic epidermal necrolysis: US FDA recommendations. Pharmacogenomics 2008;9:1543–6.
12. Miller JW. Of race, ethnicity, and rash: the genetics of antiepileptic drug-induced skin reactions. Epilepsy Curr 2008;8:120–1.
13. Locharernkul C, Loplumlert J, Limotai C. Carbamazepine and phenytoin induced Stevens-Johnson syndrome is associated with HLA-B*1502 allele in Thai population. Epilepsia 2008;49:2087–91.
14. Persson H, Ericson M, Tomson T. Carbamazepine affects autonomic cardiac control in patients with newly diagnosed epilepsy. Epilepsy Res 2003;57:69–75.
15. Saetre E, Abdelnoor M, Amlie JP, Tossebro M, Perucca E et al. Cardiac function and antiepileptic drug treatment in the elderly: A comparison between lamotrigine and sustained-release carbamazepine. Epilepsia 2009, in press.
16. Morrow J. The XX factor. Treating women with anti-epileptic drugs. Cressing, Essex: National Services for Health Improvement, 2007.
17. Morrow J, Russell A, Guthrie E, Parsons L, Robertson I, Waddell R, et al. Malformation risks of antiepileptic drugs in pregnancy: a prospective study from the UK Epilepsy and Pregnancy Register. J Neurol Neurosurg Psychiatry 2006;77:193–8.
18. Patsalos PN. Anti-epileptic drug interactions: A clinical guide. Cranleigh, UK: Clarius Press Ltd, 2005.
19. Patsalos PN, Perucca E. Clinically important drug interactions in epilepsy: general features and interactions between antiepileptic drugs. Lancet Neurol 2003;2:347–56.
20. Patsalos PN, Perucca E. Clinically important drug interactions in epilepsy: interactions between antiepileptic drugs and other drugs. Lancet Neurol 2003;2:473–81.
21. Chaves J, Sander JW. Seizure aggravation in idiopathic generalized epilepsies. Epilepsia 2005;46 Suppl 9:133–9.
22. Genton P, Gelisse P, Thomas P, Dravet C. Do carbamazepine and phenytoin aggravate juvenile myoclonic epilepsy? Neurology 2000;55:1106–9.
23. Parker AP, Agathonikou A, Robinson RO, Panayiotopoulos CP. Inappropriate use of carbamazepine and vigabatrin in typical absence seizures. Dev Med Child Neurol 1998;40:517–9.
24. Kikumoto K, Yoshinaga H, Oka M, Ito M, Endoh F, Akiyama T, et al. EEG and seizure exacerbation induced by carbamazepine in Panayiotopoulos syndrome. Epileptic Disord 2006;8:53–6.
25. Bawden HN, Camfield CS, Camfield PR, Cunningham C, Darwish H, Dooley JM, et al. The cognitive and behavioural effects of clobazam and standard monotherapy are comparable. Canadian Study Group for Childhood Epilepsy. Epilepsy Res 1999;33:133–43.

26. Mehndiratta MM, Krishnamurthy M, Rajesh KN, Singh G. Clobazam monotherapy in drug naive adult patients with epilepsy. Seizure 2003;12:226–8.
27. Montenegro MA, Ferreira CM, Cendes F, Li LM, Guerreiro CA. Clobazam as add-on therapy for temporal lobe epilepsy and hippocampal sclerosis. Can J Neurol Sci 2005;32:93–6.
28. Ng YT, Collins SD. Clobazam. Neurother 2007;4:138–44.
29. Silva RC, Montenegro MA, Guerreiro CA, Guerreiro MM. Clobazam as add-on therapy in children with epileptic encephalopathy. Can J Neurol Sci 2006;33:209–13.
30. Sugai K. Clobazam as a new antiepileptic drug and clorazepate dipotassium as an alternative antiepileptic drug in Japan. Epilepsia 2004;45 Suppl 8:20–5.
31. Conry JA, Ng YT, Paolicchi JM et al. Clobazam in the treatment of Lennox-Gastaut syndrome. Epilepsia 2009;50:1158–66.
32. Montenegro MA, Arif H, Nahm EA, Resor SR, Jr., Hirsch LJ. Efficacy of clobazam as add-on therapy for refractory epilepsy: experience at a US epilepsy center. Clin Neuropharmacol 2008;31:333–8.
33. Seo T, Nagata R, Ishitsu T. Impact of CYP2C19 polymorphisms on the efficacy of clobazam therapy. Pharmacogenomics 2008;9:527–37.
34. Clobazam has equivalent efficacy to carbamazepine and phenytoin as monotherapy for childhood epilepsy. Canadian Study Group for Childhood Epilepsy. Epilepsia 1998;39:952–9.
35. Feely M, Gibson J. Intermittent clobazam for catamenial epilepsy: tolerance avoided. J Neurol Neurosurg Psychiatry 1984;47:1279–82.
36. Parmeggiani A, Posar A, Sangiorgi S, Giovanardi-Rossi P. Unusual side effects due to clobazam: a case report with genetic study of CYP2C19. Brain Dev 2004;26:63–6.
37. Barcs G, Halasz P. Effectiveness and tolerance of clobazam in temporal lobe epilepsy. Acta Neurol Scand 1996;93:88–93.
38. Uhlmann C, Froscher W. Low risk of development of substance dependence for barbiturates and clobazam prescribed as antiepileptic drugs: results from a questionnaire study. CNS Neurosci Ther 2009;15:24–31.
39. Remy C. Clobazam in the treatment of epilepsy: a review of the literature. Epilepsia 1994;35 Suppl 5:S88–91.
40. Camfield P, Camfield C. Benzodiazepines used primarily for chronic treatment (clobazam, clonazepam, clorazepate and nitrazepam). In: Shorvon S, Perucca E, Engel JJr, eds. The treatment of epilepsy, 3nd edition, pp 421–30. Oxford: Willey-Blackwell, 2009.
41. Naito H, Wachi M, Nishida M. Clinical effects and plasma concentrations of long-term clonazepam monotherapy in previously untreated epileptics. Acta Neurol Scand 1987;76:58–63.
42. Obeid T, Panayiotopoulos CP. Clonazepam in juvenile myoclonic epilepsy. Epilepsia 1989;30:603–6.
43. Elger C, Halasz P, Maia J, Almeida L, Soares-da-Silva P. Efficacy and safety of eslicarbazepine acetate as adjunctive treatment in adults with refractory partial-onset seizures: a randomized, double-blind, placebo-controlled, parallel-group phase III study. Epilepsia 2009;50:454–63.
44. McCormack PL, Robinson DM. Eslicarbazepine acetate. CNS Drugs 2009;23:71–9.
45. Mestre T, Ferreira J. Eslicarbazepine acetate: a new option for the treatment of focal epilepsy. Expert Opin Investig Drugs 2009;18:221–9.
46. Goren MZ, Onat F. Ethosuximide: from bench to bedside. CNS Drug Rev 2007;13:224–39.
47. Posner E, Mohamed K, Marson A. Ethosuximide, sodium valproate or lamotrigine for absence seizures in children and adolescents. Cochrane Database Syst Rev 2005;CD003032.
48. Glauser TA, Perucca E. Ethosuximide. In: Shorvon S, Perucca E, Engel JJr, eds. The treatment of epilepsy, 3nd edition, pp. 499–509. Oxford: Willey-Blackwell, 2009.
49. Scott DF. The history of epileptic therapy. An account of how medication was developed. Lancashire, UK: Parthenon Publishing Group, 1993.
50. Oguni H, Uehara T, Tanaka T, Sunahara M, Hara M, Osawa M. Dramatic effect of ethosuximide on epileptic negative myoclonus: implications for the neurophysiological mechanism. Neuropediatrics 1998;29:29–34.
51. Snead OC, III, Hosey LC. Treatment of epileptic falling spells with ethosuximide. Brain Dev 1987;9:602–4.
52. Wallace SJ. Myoclonus and epilepsy in childhood: a review of treatment with valproate, ethosuximide, lamotrigine and zonisamide. Epilepsy Res 1998;29:147–54.
53. Schmitt B, Kovacevic-Preradovic T, Critelli H, Molinari L. Is ethosuximide a risk factor for generalised tonic-clonic seizures in absence epilepsy? Neuropediatrics 2007;38:83–7.
54. Coulter DA. Antiepileptic drug cellular mechanisms of action: where does lamotrigine fit in? J Child Neurol 1997;12 Suppl 1:S2–9.
55. Manning JP, Richards DA, Leresche N, Crunelli V, Bowery NG. Cortical-area specific block of genetically determined absence seizures by ethosuximide. Neuroscience 2004;123:5–9.
56. White JR, Leppik IE, Beattie JL et al. Long-term use of felbamate: Clinical outcomes and effect of age and concomitant antiepileptic drug use on its clearance. Epilepsia 2009 (in press).
57. Pellock JM, Faught E, Leppik IE, Shinnar S, Zupanc ML. Felbamate: consensus of current clinical experience. Epilepsy Res 2006;71:89–101.

58. French J, Smith M, Faught E, Brown L. Practice advisory: The use of felbamate in the treatment of patients with intractable epilepsy: report of the Quality Standards Subcommittee of the American Academy of Neurology and the American Epilepsy Society. Neurology 1999;52:1540–5.
59. Bourgeois BF. Felbamate. Semin Pediatr Neurol 1997;4:3–8.
60. Palmer KJ, McTavish D. Felbamate. A review of its pharmacodynamic and pharmacokinetic properties, and therapeutic efficacy in epilepsy. Drugs 1993;45:1041–65.
61. Battino D, Estienne M, Avanzini G. Clinical pharmacokinetics of antiepileptic drugs in paediatric patients. Part II. Phenytoin, carbamazepine, sulthiame, lamotrigine, vigabatrin, oxcarbazepine and felbamate. Clin Pharmacokinet 1995;29:341–69.
62. Pellock JM. Felbamate. Epilepsia 1999; 40 Suppl 5: S57-S62.
63. Leppik IE, White JR. Felbamate. In: Shorvon S, Perucca E, Engel JJr, eds. The treatment of epilepsy, 3nd edition, pp 511–8. Oxford: Willey-Blackwell, 2009.
64. Hussein G, Troupin AS, Montouris G. Gabapentin interaction with felbamate. Neurology 1996;47:1106.
65. Morris GL. Gabapentin. Epilepsia 1999;40 Suppl 5:S63–70.
66. McLean MJ, Gidal BE. Gabapentin dosing in the treatment of epilepsy. Clin Ther 2003;25:1382–406.
67. Shorvon SD. The choice of drugs and approach to drug treatments in partial epilepsy. In: Shorvon S, Perucca E, Fish D, Dodson E, eds. The treatment of epilepsy. Second edition, pp 317–33. Oxford: Blackwell Publishing, 2004.
68. Chadwick D, Leiderman DB, Sauermann W, Alexander J, Garofalo E. Gabapentin in generalized seizures. Epilepsy Res 1996;25:191–7.
69. Thomas P, Valton L, Genton P. Absence and myoclonic status epilepticus precipitated by antiepileptic drugs in idiopathic generalized epilepsy. Brain 2006;129 Pt 5:1281–92.
70. Striano P, Coppola A, Madia F, Pezzella M, Ciampa C et al. Life-threatening status epilepticus following gabapentin administration in a patient with benign adult familial myoclonic epilepsy. Epilepsia 2007;48:1995–8.
71. Tomson T, Dahl M, Kimland E. Therapeutic monitoring of antiepileptic drugs for epilepsy. Cochrane Database Syst Rev 2007;(1):CD002216.
72. Johannessen SI, Tomson T. Pharmacokinetic variability of newer antiepileptic drugs: when is monitoring needed? Clin Pharmacokinet 2006;45:1061–75.
73. Wolf SM, Shinnar S, Kang H, Gil KB, Moshe SL. Gabapentin toxicity in children manifesting as behavioral changes. Epilepsia 1995;36:1203–5.
74. Boneva N, Brenner T, Argov Z. Gabapentin may be hazardous in myasthenia gravis. Muscle Nerve 2000;23:1204–8.
75. Prakash, Prabhu LV, Rai R, Pai MM, Yadav SK, Madhyastha S et al. Teratogenic effects of the anticonvulsant gabapentin in mice. Singapore Med J 2008;49:47–53.
76. Beydoun A, D'Souza J, Hebert D, Doty P. Lacosamide: pharmacology, mechanisms of action and pooled efficacy and safety data in partial-onset seizures. Expert Rev Neurother 2009;9:33–42.
77. Curia G, Biagini G, Perucca E, Avoli M. Lacosamide: a new approach to target voltage-gated sodium currents in epileptic disorders. CNS Drugs 2009;23:555–68.
78. Halford JJ, Lapointe M. Clinical perspectives on lacosamide. Epilepsy Curr 2009;9:1–9.
79. Kellinghaus C, Berning S, Besselmann M. Intravenous lacosamide as successful treatment for nonconvulsive status epilepticus after failure of first-line therapy. Epilepsy Behav 2009 (in press).
80. Biton V. Lacosamide. In: Panayiotopoulos CP, ed. Atlas of epilepsies. London: Springer, 2010 (in press).
81. Biton V, Rosenfeld WE, Whitesides J, Fountain NB, Vaiciene N, Rudd GD. Intravenous lacosamide as replacement for oral lacosamide in patients with partial-onset seizures. Epilepsia 2008;49:418–24.
82. Errington AC, Stohr T, Heers C, Lees G. The investigational anticonvulsant lacosamide selectively enhances slow inactivation of voltage-gated sodium channels. Mol Pharmacol 2008;73:157–69.
83. Perucca E, Yasothan U, Clincke G, Kirkpatrick P. Lacosamide. Nat Rev Drug Discov 2008;7:973–4.
84. Cross SA, Curran MP. Lacosamide: in partial-onset seizures. Drugs 2009;69:449-59.
85. Barron TF, Hunt SL, Hoban TF, Price ML. Lamotrigine monotherapy in children. Pediatr Neurol 2000;23:160–3.
86. Culy CR, Goa KL. Lamotrigine. A review of its use in childhood epilepsy. Paediatr Drugs 2000;2:299–330.
87. Messenheimer J, Mullens EL, Giorgi L, Young F. Safety review of adult clinical trial experience with lamotrigine. Drug Saf 1998;18:281–96.
88. Mullens EL. Lamotrigine monotherapy in epilepsy. Clin Drug Invest 1998;16:125–33.
89. Brodie MJ. Lamotrigine – an update. Can J Neurol Sci 1996;23:S6–9.
90. Messenheimer JA. Lamotrigine. Epilepsia 1995;36 Suppl 2:S87–94.
91. Faught E. Lamotrigine for startle-induced seizures. Seizure 1999;8:361–3.
92. Frank LM, Enlow T, Holmes GL, Manasco P, Concannon S, Chen C, et al. Lamictal (lamotrigine) monotherapy for typical absence seizures in children. Epilepsia 1999;40:973–9.
93. Barr PA, Buettiker VE, Antony JH. Efficacy of lamotrigine in refractory neonatal seizures. Pediatr Neurol 1999;20:161–3.

94. Gamble C, Williamson PR, Chadwick DW, Marson AG. A meta-analysis of individual patient responses to lamotrigine or carbamazepine monotherapy. Neurology 2006;66:1310–7.

95. Marson AG, Al-Kharusi AM, Alwaidh M, Appleton R, Baker GA, Chadwick DW, et al. The SANAD study of eff ectiveness of carbamazepine, gabapentin, lamotrigine, oxcarbazepine, or topiramate for treatment of partial epilepsy: an unblinded randomised controlled trial. Lancet 2007:369:1000–15.

96. French JA, Kryscio RJ. Active control trials for epilepsy. Avoiding bias in head-to-head trials. Neurology 2006;66:1294–5.

97. French JA. First-choice drug for newly diagnosed epilepsy. Lancet 2007;369:970–1.

98. French J. Can evidence-based guidelines and clinical trials tell us how to treat patients? Epilepsia 2007; 48:1264–1267.

99. Panayiotopoulos CP. Evidence-based epileptology, randomised controlled trials, and SANAD: A critical clinical view. Epilepsia 2007; 48:1268–1274.

100. Panayiotopoulos CP, Ferrie CD, Knott C, Robinson RO. Interaction of lamotrigine with sodium valproate. Lancet 1993;341:445.

101. Ferrie CD, Panayiotopoulos CP. Therapeutic interaction of lamotrigine and sodium valproate in intractable myoclonic epilepsy. Seizure 1994;3:157–9.

102. Mikati MA, Holmes GL. Lamotrigine in absence and primary generalized epilepsies. J Child Neurol 1997;12 Suppl 1:S29–37.

103. Brodie MJ, Yuen AW. Lamotrigine substitution study: evidence for synergism with sodium valproate? 105 Study Group. Epilepsy Res 1997;26:423–32.

104. Pressler RM, Binnie CD, Coleshill SG, Chorley GA, Robinson RO. Effect of lamotrigine on cognition in children with epilepsy. Neurology 2006;66:1495–9.

105. Blum D, Meador K, Biton V, Fakhoury T, Shneker B, Chung S, et al. Cognitive effects of lamotrigine compared with topiramate in patients with epilepsy. Neurology 2006;67:400–6.

106. Labiner DM, Ettinger AB, Fakhoury TA, Chung SS, Shneker B, Tatumlv WO et al. Effects of lamotrigine compared with levetiracetam on anger, hostility, and total mood in patients with partial epilepsy. Epilepsia 2009;50:434–42.

107. Faught E, Morris G, Jacobson M, French J, Harden C, Montouris G, et al. Adding lamotrigine to valproate: incidence of rash and other adverse effects. Postmarketing Antiepileptic Drug Survey (PADS) Group. Epilepsia 1999;40:1135–40.

108. Guberman AH, Besag FM, Brodie MJ, Dooley JM, Duchowny MS, Pellock JM, et al. Lamotrigine-associated rash: risk/benefit considerations in adults and children. Epilepsia 1999;40:985–91.

109. Hirsch LJ, Weintraub DB, Buchsbaum R, Spencer HT, Straka T, Hager M, et al. Predictors of lamotrigine-associated rash. Epilepsia 2006;47:318–22.

110. Steinhoff BJ. How to replace lamotrigine with valproate. Epilepsia 2006;47:1943–4

111. Patsalos PN, Berry DJ, Bourgeois BF, Cloyd JC, Glauser TA, Johannessen SI et al. Antiepileptic drugs--best practice guidelines for therapeutic drug monitoring: a position paper by the subcommission on therapeutic drug monitoring, ILAE Commission on Therapeutic Strategies. Epilepsia 2008;49:1239–76.

112. Tran TA, Leppik IE, Blesi K, Sathanandan ST, Remmel R. Lamotrigine clearance during pregnancy. Neurology 2002;59:251–5.

113. de Haan GJ, Edelbroek P, Segers J, Engelsman M, Lindhout D, Devile-Notschaele M, et al. Gestation-induced changes in lamotrigine pharmacokinetics: a monotherapy study. Neurology 2004;63:571–3.

114. Pennell PB, Newport DJ, Stowe ZN, Helmers SL, Montgomery JQ, Henry TR. The impact of pregnancy and childbirth on the metabolism of lamotrigine. Neurology 2004;62:292–5.

115. Sabers A, Ohman I, Christensen J, Tomson T. Oral contraceptives reduce lamotrigine plasma levels. Neurology 2003;61:570–1.

116. Paul F, Veauthier C, Fritz G, Lehmann TN, Aktas O, Zipp F, et al. Perioperative fluctuations of lamotrigine serum levels in patients undergoing epilepsy surgery. Seizure 2007; In press.

117. Aurlien D, Tauboll E, Gjerstad L. Lamotrigine in idiopathic epilepsy – increased risk of cardiac death? Acta Neurol Scand 2007;115:199–203.

118. Van Landingham KE, Dixon RM. Lamotrigine in idiopathic epilepsy - increased risk of cardiac death. Acta Neurol Scand 2007;116:345.

119. Aurlien D, Tauboll E, Gjerstad L. An insufficient effect of lamotrigine leading to fatal seizures. Acta Neurol Scand 2008;117:293.

120. Dixon R, Job S, Oliver R, Tompson D, Wright JG, Maltby K et al. Lamotrigine does not prolong QTc in a thorough QT/QTc study in healthy subjects. Br J Clin Pharmacol 2008;66:396–404.

121. Saetre E, Abdelnoor M, Amlie JP, Tossebro M, Perucca E, Taubøll E et al. Cardiac function and antiepileptic drug treatment in the elderly: A comparison between lamotrigine and sustained-release carbamazepine. Epilepsia 2009, in press.

122. Holmes LB, Baldwin EJ, Smith CR, Habecker E, Glassman L, Wong SL et al. Increased frequency of isolated cleft palate in infants exposed to lamotrigine during pregnancy. Neurology 2008;70:2152–2158.

123. Hunt SJ, Craig JJ, Morrow JI. Increased frequency of isolated cleft palate in infants exposed to lamotrigine during pregnancy. Neurology 2009;72:1108–9.
124. Cunnington M, Tennis P. Lamotrigine and the risk of malformations in pregnancy. Neurology 2005;64:955–60.
125. Tomson T, Luef G, Sabers A, Pittschieler S, Ohman I. Valproate effects on kinetics of lamotrigine in pregnancy and treatment with oral contraceptives. Neurology 2006;67:1297–9.
126. Zupanc ML. Antiepileptic drugs and hormonal contraceptives in adolescent women with epilepsy. Neurology 2006;66 Suppl 3:S37–45.
127. Dubnov-Raz G, Shapiro R, Merlob P. Maternal lamotrigine treatment and elevated neonatal gamma-glutamyl transpeptidase. Pediatr Neurol 2006;35:220–2.
128. Fitton A, Goa KL. Lamotrigine. An update of its pharmacology and therapeutic use in epilepsy. Drugs 1995;50:691–713.
129. Seizure control and treatment in pregnancy: observations from the EURAP epilepsy pregnancy registry. Neurology 2006;66:354–60.
130. Carrazana EJ, Wheeler SD. Exacerbation of juvenile myoclonic epilepsy with lamotrigine. Neurology 2001;56:1424–5.
131. Biraben A, Allain H, Scarabin JM, Schuck S, Edan G. Exacerbation of juvenile myoclonic epilepsy with lamotrigine. Neurology 2000;55:1758.
132. Maiga Y, Nogues B, Guillon B. [Exacerbation of tonicoclonic seizures in a juvenile myoclonic epileptic taking lamotrigine.] Rev Neurol (Paris) 2006;162:1125–7.
133. Guerrini R, Dravet C, Genton P, Belmonte A, Kaminska A, Dulac O. Lamotrigine and seizure aggravation in severe myoclonic epilepsy. Epilepsia 1998;39:508–12.
134. Guerrini R, Belmonte A, Parmeggiani L, Perucca E. Myoclonic status epilepticus following high-dosage lamotrigine therapy. Brain Dev 1999;21:420–4.
135. Genton P, Gelisse P, Crespel A. Lack of efficacy and potential aggravation of myoclonus with lamotrigine in Unverricht-Lundborg disease. Epilepsia 2006;47:2083–5.
136. Abou-Khalil B. Levetiracetam in the treatment of epilepsy. Neuropsychiatr Dis Treat 2008;4:507–23.
137. Glauser TA, Pellock JM, Bebin EM, Fountain NB, Ritter FJ, Jensen CM, et al. Efficacy and safety of levetiracetam in children with partial seizures: an open-label trial. Epilepsia 2002;43:518–24.
138. Kaminski RM, Matagne A, Patsalos PN, Klitgaard H. Benefit of combination therapy in epilepsy: a review of the preclinical evidence with levetiracetam. Epilepsia 2009;50:387–97.
139. Peltola J, Coetzee C, Jimenez F, Litovchenko T, Ramaratnam S, Zaslavaskiy L et al. Once-daily extended-release levetiracetam as adjunctive treatment of partial-onset seizures in patients with epilepsy: a double-blind, randomized, placebo-controlled trial. Epilepsia 2009;50:406–14.
140. Morrell MJ, Leppik I, French J, Ferrendelli J, Han J, Magnus L. The KEEPER trial: levetiracetam adjunctive treatment of partial-onset seizures in an open-label community-based study. Epilepsy Res 2003;54:153–61.
141. Ferrendelli JA, French J, Leppik I, Morrell MJ, Herbeuval A, Han J, et al. Use of levetiracetam in a population of patients aged 65 years and older: a subset analysis of the KEEPER trial. Epilepsy Behav 2003;4:702–9.
142. French JA, Tonner F. Levetiracetam. In: Shorvon S, Perucca E, Engel JJr, eds. The treatment of epilepsy (3nd edition). Oxford: Willey-Blackwell, 2009:559–73.
143. Briggs DE, French JA. Levetiracetam safety profiles and tolerability in epilepsy patients. Expert Opin Drug Saf 2004;3:415–24.
144. Patsalos PN. Levetiracetam. Rev Contemp Pharmacol 2004;13:1–168.
145. Cramer JA, Arrigo C, Van Hammee G, Gauer LJ, Cereghino JJ. Effect of levetiracetam on epilepsy-related quality of life. N132 Study Group. Epilepsia 2000;41:868–74.
146. Marson AG, Hutton JL, Leach JP, Castillo S, Schmidt D, White S, et al. Levetiracetam, oxcarbazepine, remacemide and zonisamide for drug resistant localization-related epilepsy: a systematic review. Epilepsy Res 2001;46:259–70.
147. Ben Menachem E. Preliminary efficacy of levetiracetam in monotherapy. Epileptic Disord 2003;5 Suppl 1:S51–5.
148. Patsalos PN. Properties of antiepileptic drugs in the treatment of idiopathic generalized epilepsies. Epilepsia 2005;46 Suppl 9:140–8.
149. Specchio LM, Boero G, Specchio N, De Agazio G, De Palo A, de Tommaso M, et al. Evidence for a rapid action of levetiracetam compared to topiramate in refractory partial epilepsy. Seizure 2006;15:112–6.
150. Stefan H, Wang-Tilz Y, Pauli E, Dennhofer S, Genow A, Kerling F, et al. Onset of action of levetiracetam: a RCT trial using therapeutic intensive seizure analysis (TISA). Epilepsia 2006;47:516–22.
151. Perucca E, Johannessen SI. The ideal pharmacokinetic properties of an antiepileptic drug: how close does levetiracetam come? Epileptic Disord 2003;5 Suppl 1:S17–26.
152. Privitera M. Efficacy of levetiracetam: a review of three pivotal clinical trials. Epilepsia 2001;42 Suppl 4:31–5.
153. Chaisewikul R, Privitera MD, Hutton JL, Marson AG. Levetiracetam add-on for drug-resistant localization related (partial) epilepsy. Cochrane Database Syst Rev 2001;1:CD001901.
154. Beran RG, Berkovic SF, Black AB, Danta G, Hiersemenzel R, Schapel GJ, et al. Efficacy and safety of levetiracetam 1000–3000 mg/day in patients with refractory partial-onset seizures: a multicenter, open-label single-arm study. Epilepsy Res 2005;63:1–9.

155. Abou-Khalil B. Benefit-risk assessment of levetiracetam in the treatment of partial seizures. Drug Saf 2005;28:871–90.
156. Otoul C, Arrigo C, van Rijckevorsel K, French JA. Meta-analysis and indirect comparisons of levetiracetam with other second generation antiepileptic drugs in partial epilepsy. Clin Neuropharmacol 2005;28:72–8.
157. Genton P, Sadzot B, Fejerman N, Peltola J, Despland PA, Steinhoff B, et al. Levetiracetam in a broad population of patients with refractory epilepsy: interim results of the international SKATE trial. Acta Neurol Scand 2006;113:387–94.
158. Leppik I, De RK, Edrich P, Perucca E. Measurement of seizure freedom in adjunctive therapy studies in refractory partial epilepsy: the levetiracetam experience. Epileptic Disord 2006;8:118–30.
159. Lambrechts DA, Sadzot B, Van PW, van Leusden JA, Carpay J, Bourgeois P, et al. Efficacy and safety of levetiracetam in clinical practice: results of the SKATE trial from Belgium and The Netherlands. Seizure 2006;15:434–42.
160. Bauer J, Ben-Menachem E, Kramer G, Fryze W, Da SS, Kasteleijn- Nolst Trenite DG. Levetiracetam: a long-term follow-up study of efficacy and safety. Acta Neurol Scand 2006;114:169–76.
161. Brodie MJ, Perucca E, Ryvlin P, Ben-Menachem E, Meencke HJ; Levetiracetam Monotherapy Study Group. Comparison of levetiracetam and controlled-release carbamazepine in newly diagnosed epilepsy. Neurology 2007;68:402–8.
162. Peake D, Mordekar S, Gosalakkal J, Mukhtyar B, Buch S, Crane J, et al. Retention rate of levetiracetam in children with intractable epilepsy at 1 year. Seizure 2007;16:185–9.
163. Noachtar S, Andermann E, Meyvisch P, Andermann F, Gough WB, Schiemann-Delgado J. Levetiracetam for the treatment of idiopathic generalized epilepsy with myoclonic seizures. Neurology 2008;70:607–16.
164. Berkovic SF, Knowlton RC, Leroy RF, Schiemann J, Falter U. Placebo-controlled study of levetiracetam in idiopathic generalized epilepsy. Neurology 2007;69:1751–60.
165. Sharpe DV, Patel AD, Abou-Khalil B, Fenichel GM. Levetiracetam monotherapy in juvenile myoclonic epilepsy. Seizure 2008;17:64–8.
166. Verrotti A, Cerminara C, Coppola G, Franzoni E, Parisi P, Iannetti P et al. Levetiracetam in juvenile myoclonic epilepsy: long-term efficacy in newly diagnosed adolescents. Dev Med Child Neurol 2008;50:29–32.
167. Verrotti A, Cerminara C, Domizio S, Mohn A, Franzoni E, Coppola G et al. Levetiracetam in absence epilepsy. Dev Med Child Neurol 2008;50:850-3.
168. Coppola G, Franzoni E, Verrotti A, Garone C, Sarajlija J, Felicia OF, et al. Levetiracetam or oxcarbazepine as monotherapy in newly diagnosed benign epilepsy of childhood with centrotemporal spikes (BECTS): An open-label, parallel group trial. Brain Dev 2007;29:281–4.
169. Verrotti A, Coppola G, Manco R, Ciambra G, Iannetti P, Grosso S, et al. Levetiracetam monotherapy for children and adolescents with benign rolandic seizures. Seizure 2007;16:271–5.
170. Bello-Espinosa LE, Roberts SL. Levetiracetam for benign epilepsy of childhood with centrotemporal spikes – three cases. Seizure 2003;12:157–9.
171. Huber B, Bommel W, Hauser I, Horstmann V, Liem S, May T, et al. Efficacy and tolerability of levetiracetam in patients with therapy resistant epilepsy and learning disabilities. Seizure 2004;13:168–75.
172. Wang SB, Weng WC, Fan PC, Lee WT. Levetiracetam in continuous spike waves during slow-wave sleep syndrome. Pediatr Neurol 2008;39:85–90.
173. Kossoff EH, Boatman D, Freeman JM. Landau-Kleffner syndrome responsive to levetiracetam. Epilepsy Behav 2003;4:571–5.
174. Labate A, Colosimo E, Gambardella A, Leggio U, Ambrosio R, Quattrone A. Levetiracetam in patients with generalised epilepsy and myoclonic seizures: an open label study. Seizure 2006;15:214–8.
175. Maschio M, Albani F, Baruzzi A, Zarabla A, Dinapoli L, Pace A, et al. Levetiracetam therapy in patients with brain tumour and epilepsy. J Neurooncol 2006;80:97–100.
176. Newton HB, Goldlust SA, Pearl D. Retrospective analysis of the efficacy and tolerability of levetiracetam in brain tumor patients. J Neurooncol 2006;78:99–102.
177. Alsaadi TM, Koopmans S, Apperson M, Farias S. Levetiracetam monotherapy for elderly patients with epilepsy. Seizure 2004;13:58–60.
178. Cramer JA, Leppik IE, Rue KD, Edrich P, Kramer G. Tolerability of levetiracetam in elderly patients with CNS disorders. Epilepsy Res 2003;56:135–45.
179. Baulac M, Brodie MJ, Elger CE, Krakow K, Stockis A, Meyvisch P, et al. Levetiracetam intravenous infusion as an alternative to oral dosing in patients with partial-onset seizures. Epilepsia 2007;48:589–92.
180. Pina-Garza JE, Nordli DR, Jr., Rating D, Yang H, Schiemann-Delgado J, Duncan B. Adjunctive levetiracetam in infants and young children with refractory partial-onset seizures. Epilepsia 2009;50:1141–9.
181. Tan MJ, Appleton RE. Efficacy and tolerability of levetiracetam in children aged 10 years and younger: a clinical experience. Seizure 2004;13:142–5.
182. Wheless JW, Ng YT. Levetiracetam in refractory pediatric epilepsy. J Child Neurol 2002;17:413–5.
183. Lagae L, Buyse G, Deconinck A, Ceulemans B. Effect of levetiracetam in refractory childhood epilepsy syndromes. Eur J Paediatr Neurol 2003;7:123–8.
184. French J. Use of levetiracetam in special populations. Epilepsia 2001;42 Suppl 4:40–3.

185. Pellock JM, Glauser TA, Bebin EM, Fountain NB, Ritter FJ, Coupez RM, et al. Pharmacokinetic study of levetiracetam in children. Epilepsia 2001;42:1574–9.
186. Glauser TA, Dulac O. Preliminary efficacy of levetiracetam in children. Epileptic Disord 2003;5 Suppl 1:S45–50.
187. Glauser TA, Mitchell WG, Weinstock A, Bebin M, Chen D, Coupez R, et al. Pharmacokinetics of levetiracetam in infants and young children with epilepsy. Epilepsia 2007;48:1117–22.
188. Ramael S, De SF, Toublanc N, Otoul C, Boulanger P, Riethuisen JM, et al. Single-dose bioavailability of levetiracetam intravenous infusion relative to oral tablets and multiple-dose pharmacokinetics and tolerability of levetiracetam intravenous infusion compared with placebo in healthy subjects. Clin Ther 2006;28:734–44.
189. Ramael S, Daoust A, Otoul C, Toublanc N, Troenaru M, Lu ZS, et al. Levetiracetam intravenous infusion: a randomized, placebo-controlled safety and pharmacokinetic study. Epilepsia 2006;47:1128–35.
190. Tomson T, Palm R, Kallen K, Ben-Menachem E, Soderfeldt B, Danielsson B, et al. Pharmacokinetics of levetiracetam during pregnancy, delivery, in the neonatal period, and lactation. Epilepsia 2007;48:1111–6.
191. French J, Edrich P, Cramer JA. A systematic review of the safety profile of levetiracetam: a new antiepileptic drug. Epilepsy Res 2001;47:77–90.
192. Sohn YH, Jung HY, Kaelin-Lang A, Hallett M. Effect of levetiracetam on rapid motor learning in humans. Arch Neurol 2002;59:1909–1912.
193. Nakken KO, Eriksson AS, Lossius R, Johannessen SI. A paradoxical effect of levetiracetam may be seen in both children and adults with refractory epilepsy. Seizure 2003;12:42–6.
194. Hunt S, Craig J, Russell A, Guthrie E, Parsons L, Robertson I, et al. Levetiracetam in pregnancy: preliminary experience from the UK Epilepsy and Pregnancy Register. Neurology 2006;67:1876–9.
195. Johannessen SI, Helde G, Brodtkorb E. Levetiracetam concentrations in serum and in breast milk at birth and during lactation. Epilepsia 2005;46:775–7.
196. Klitgaard H, Pitkanen A. Antiepileptogenesis, neuroprotection, and disease modification in the treatment of epilepsy: focus on levetiracetam. Epileptic Disord 2003;5 Suppl 1:S9–16.
197. Klitgaard H, Matagne A, Gobert J, Wulfert E. Evidence for a unique profile of levetiracetam in rodent models of seizures and epilepsy. Eur J Pharmacol 1998;353:191–206.
198. Klitgaard H. Levetiracetam: the preclinical profile of a new class of antiepileptic drugs? Epilepsia 2001;42 Suppl 4:13–8.
199. Lynch BA, Lambeng N, Nocka K, Kensel-Hammes P, Bajjalieh SM, Matagne A, et al. The synaptic vesicle protein SV2A is the binding site for the antiepileptic drug levetiracetam. Proc Natl Acad Sci USA 2004;101:9861–6.
200. Gillard M, Chatelain P, Fuks B. Binding characteristics of levetiracetam to synaptic vesicle protein 2A (SV2A) in human brain and in CHO cells expressing the human recombinant protein. Eur J Pharmacol 2006;536:102–8.
201. Patsalos PN. Pharmacokinetic profile of levetiracetam: toward ideal characteristics. Pharmacol Ther 2000;85:77–85.
202. Contin M, Albani F, Riva R, Baruzzi A. Levetiracetam therapeutic monitoring in patients with epilepsy: effect of concomitant antiepileptic drugs. Ther Drug Monit 2004;26:375–9.
203. White JR, Walczak TS, Leppik IE, Rarick J, Tran T, Beniak TE, et al. Discontinuation of levetiracetam because of behavioral side effects: A case-control study. Neurology 2003;61:1218–21.
204. Mula M, Trimble MR, Sander JW. Psychiatric adverse events in patients with epilepsy and learning disabilities taking levetiracetam. Seizure 2004;13:55–7.
205. Hurtado B, Koepp MJ, Sander JW, Thompson PJ. The impact of levetiracetam on challenging behavior. Epilepsy Behav 2006;8:588–92.
206. Weintraub D, Buchsbaum R, Resor SR, Jr, Hirsch LJ. Psychiatric and behavioral side effects of the newer antiepileptic drugs in adults with epilepsy. Epilepsy Behav 2007;10:105–10.
207. Ciesielski AS, Samson S, Steinhoff BJ. Neuropsychological and psychiatric impact of add-on titration of pregabalin versus levetiracetam: a comparative short-term study. Epilepsy Behav 2006;9:424–31.
208. Schmidt D, Elger CE. What is the evidence that oxcarbazepine and carbamazepine are distinctly different antiepileptic drugs? Epilepsy Behav 2004;5:627–35.
209. Bang LM, Goa KL. Spotlight on oxcarbazepine in epilepsy. CNS Drugs 2004;18:57–61.
210. Faught E, Limdi N. Oxcarbazepine. In: Shorvon S, Perucca E, Engel JJr, eds. The treatment of epilepsy, 3nd edition, pp 575–84. Oxford: Willey-Blackwell, 2009.
211. Muller M, Marson AG, Williamson PR. Oxcarbazepine versus phenytoin monotherapy for epilepsy. Cochrane Database Syst Rev 2006;(2):CD003615.
212. Christensen J, Sabers A, Sidenius P. Oxcarbazepine concentrations during pregnancy: a retrospective study in patients with epilepsy. Neurology 2006;67:1497–9.
213. Mazzucchelli I, Onat FY, Ozkara C, Atakli D, Specchio LM, Neve AL, et al. Changes in the disposition of oxcarbazepine and its metabolites during pregnancy and the puerperium. Epilepsia 2006;47:504–9.
214. Gelisse P, Genton P, Kuate D, Pesenti A, Baldy-Moulinier M, Crespel A. Worsening of seizures by oxcarbazepine in juvenile idiopathic generalized epilepsies. Epilepsia 2004;45:1282–8.
215. Albani F, Grassi B, Ferrara R, Turrini R, Baruzzi A. Immediate (overnight) switching from carbamazepine to oxcarbazepine monotherapy is equivalent to a progressive switch. Seizure 2004;13:254–63.

216. Taylor S, Tudur S, Williamson PR, Marson AG. Phenobarbitone versus phenytoin monotherapy for partial onset seizures and generalized onset tonic-clonic seizures. Cochrane Database Syst Rev 2001;(4):CD002217.

217. de Silva M, MacArdle B, McGowan M, Hughes E, Stewart J, Neville BG, et al. Randomised comparative monotherapy trial of phenobarbitone, phenytoin, carbamazepine, or sodium valproate for newly diagnosed childhood epilepsy. Lancet 1996;347:709–13.

218. Heller AJ, Chesterman P, Elwes RD, Crawford P, Chadwick D, Johnson, et al. Phenobarbitone, phenytoin, carbamazepine, or sodium valproate for newly diagnosed adult epilepsy: a randomised comparative monotherapy trial. J Neurol Neurosurg Psychiatr 1995;58:44–50.

219. Michelucci R, Pasini E, Tassinari AC. Phenobarbital, primidone and other barbiturates. In: Shorvon S, Perucca E, Engel JJr, eds. The treatment of epilepsy, 3nd edition, pp 458–74. Oxford: Wiley-Blackwell, 2009:459–74.

220. Mattson RH, Cramer JA, Collins JF, Smith DB, Delgado-Escueta AV, Browne TR, et al. Comparison of carbamazepine, phenobarbital, phenytoin, and primidone in partial and secondarily generalized tonic-clonic seizures. N Engl J Med 1985;313:145–51.

221. Reis TT, Maia Filho PC, Cechini PC. [Clinical evaluation of the therapeutic value of barbexaclone including determination of plasma levels of the barbiturate]. Arq Neuropsiquiatr 1980;38:93–8.

222. Eadie MJ. Phenytoin. In: Shorvon S, Perucca E, Engel JJr, eds. The treatment of epilepsy, 3nd edition, pp 605–18. Oxford: Wiley-Blackwell, 2009.

223. Bebin M, Bleck TP. New anticonvulsant drugs. Focus on flunarizine, fosphenytoin, midazolam and stiripentol. Drugs 1994;48:153–171.

224. Pellock JM. Fosphenytoin use in children. Neurology 1996;46 Suppl 1:S14–6.

225. Browne TR. Fosphenytoin (Cerebyx). Clin Neuropharmacol 1997;20:1–12.

226. Voytko SM, Farrington E. Fosphenytoin sodium: new drug to replace intravenous phenytoin sodium. Pediatr Nurs 1997;23:503–6.

227. Luer MS. Fosphenytoin. Neurol Res 1998;20:17882.

228. DeToledo JC, Ramsay RE. Fosphenytoin and phenytoin in patients with status epilepticus: improved tolerability versus increased costs. Drug Saf 2000;22:459–66.

229. Beydoun A, Uthman BM, Kugler AR, Greiner MJ, Knapp LE, Garofalo EA. Safety and efficacy of two pregabalin regimens for add on treatment of partial epilepsy. Neurology 2005;64:475–80.

230. Elger CE, Brodie MJ, Anhut H, Lee CM, Barrett JA. Pregabalin add on treatment in patients with partial seizures: a novel evaluation of flexible-dose and fixed-dose treatment in a double-blind, placebocontrolled study. Epilepsia 2005;46:1926–36.

231. Ryvlin P. Defining success in clinical trials – profiling pregabalin, the newest AED. Eur J Neurol 2005;12 Suppl 4:12–21.

232. Gil-Nagel A, Zaccara G, Baldinetti F, Leon T. Add-on treatment with pregabalin for partial seizures with or without generalisation: pooled data analysis of four randomised placebo-controlled trials. Seizure 2009;18:184–92.

233. Arroyo S, Anhut H, Kugler AR, Lee CM, Knapp LE, Garofalo EA, et al. Pregabalin add-on treatment: a randomized, double-blind, placebocontrolled, dose-response study in adults with partial seizures. Epilepsia 2004;45:20–7.

234. Huppertz HJ, Feuerstein TJ, Schulze-Bonhage A. Myoclonus in epilepsy patients with anticonvulsive add-on therapy with pregabalin. Epilepsia 2001;42:790–2.

235. Joshi I, Taylor CP. Pregabalin action at a model synapse: binding to presynaptic calcium channel alpha2-delta subunit reduces neurotransmission in mice. Eur J Pharmacol 2006;553:82–8.

236. Brodie MJ, Wilson EA, Wesche DL, Alvey CW, Randinitis EJ, Posvar EL, et al. Pregabalin drug interaction studies: lack of effect on the pharmacokinetics of carbamazepine, phenytoin, lamotrigine, and valproate in patients with partial epilepsy. Epilepsia 2005;46:1407–13.

237. Fink K, Dooley DJ, Meder WP, Suman-Chauhan N, Duffy S, Clusmann H, et al. Inhibition of neuronal Ca(2+) influx by gabapentin and pregabalin in the human neocortex. Neuropharmacology 2002;42:229–36.

238. Palhagen S, Canger R, Henriksen O, van Parys JA, Riviere ME, Karolchyk MA. Rufinamide: a double-blind, placebo controlled proof of principle trial in patients with epilepsy. Epilepsy Res 2001;43:115–24.

239. Biton V. Rufinamide. In: Shorvon S, Perucca E, Engel JJr, eds. The treatment of epilepsy (3nd edition). Oxford: Willey-Blackwell, 2009:647-55.

240. Cheng-Hakimian A, Anderson GD, Miller JW. Rufinamide: pharmacology, clinical trials, and role in clinical practice. Int J Clin Pract 2006;60:1497–501.

241. Deeks ED, Scott LJ. Rufinamide. CNS Drugs 2006;20:751–60.

242. Arroyo S. Rufinamide. Neurother 2007;4:155–62.

243. Moreland TA, Astoin J, Lepage F, Tombret F, Levy RH, Baillie TA. The metabolic fate of stiripentol in man. Drug Metab Dispos 1986;14:654-62.

244. Vincent JC. Stiripentol. Epilepsy Res Suppl 1991;3:153–6.

245. Perez J, Chiron C, Musial C. Stiripentol: efficacy and tolerability in children with epilepsy. Epilepsia 1999;40:1618–26.

246. Chiron C. Stiripentol. Neurother 2007;4:123–5.

247. Fisher JL. The anti-convulsant stiripentol acts directly on the GABA(A) receptor as a positive allosteric modulator. Neuropharmacology 2009;56:190–7.

248. Inoue Y, Ohtsuka Y, Oguni H, Tohyama J, Baba H, Fukushima K et al. Stiripentol open study in Japanese patients with Dravet syndrome. Epilepsia 2009 (in press).

249. Koepp MJ, Patsalos PN, Sander JW. Sulthiame in adults with refractory epilepsy and learning disability: an open trial. Epilepsy Res 2002;50:277–82.

250. Kramer U, Shahar E, Zelnik N, Lerman-Sagie T, Watemberg N, Nevo Y, et al. Carbamazepine versus sulthiame in treating benign childhood epilepsy with centrotemporal spikes. J Child Neurol 2002;17:914–6.

251. Bast T, Volp A, Wolf C, Rating D. The influence of sulthiame on EEG in children with benign childhood epilepsy with centrotemporal spikes (BECTS). Epilepsia 2003;44:215–20.

252. Engler F, Maeder-Ingvar M, Roulet E, Deonna T. Treatment with sulthiame (Ospolot) in benign partial epilepsy of childhood and related syndromes: an open clinical and EEG study. Neuropediatrics 2003;34:105–9.

253. Wirrell E, Ho AW, Hamiwka L. Sulthiame therapy for continuous spike and wave in slow-wave sleep. Pediatr Neurol 2006;35:204–8.

254. Green JR, Troupin AS, Halperm LM, Friel P, Kanarek P. Sulthiame: evaluation as an anticonvulsant. Epilepsia 1974;15:329–49.

255. Houghton GW, Richens A. Phenytoin intoxication induced by sulthiame in epileptic patients. J Neurol Neurosurg Psychiatry 1974;37:275–81.

256. Lerman P, Nussbaum E. The use of sulthiame in myoclonic epilepsy of childhood and adolescence. Acta Neurol Scand Suppl 1975;60:7–12.

257. Kalviainen R. Tiagabine. In: Shorvon S, Perucca E, Engel JJr, eds. The treatment of epilepsy (3nd edition). Oxford: Willey-Blackwell, 2009:663–72.

258. Loiseau P. Review of controlled trials of gabitril (tiagabine): a clinician's viewpoint. Epilepsia 1999;40 Suppl 9:S14–9.

259. Schmidt D, Gram L, Brodie M, Kramer G, Perucca E, Kalviainen R, et al. Tiagabine in the treatment of epilepsy – a clinical review with a guide for the prescribing physician. Epilepsy Res 2000;41:245–51.

260. Krauss GL, Johnson MA, Sheth S, Miller NR. A controlled study comparing visual function in patients treated with vigabatrin and tiagabine. J Neurol Neurosurg Psychiatry 2003;74:339–43.

261. Lawden MC. Vigabatrin, tiagabine, and visual fields. J Neurol Neurosurg Psychiatry 2003;74:286.

262. Shinnar S, Berg AT, Treiman DM, Hauser WA, Hesdorffer DC, Sackellares JC, et al. Status epilepticus and tiagabine therapy: review of safety data and epidemiologic comparisons. Epilepsia 2001;42:372–9.

263. Knake S, Hamer HM, Schomburg U, Oertel WH, Rosenow F. Tiagabine-induced absence status in idiopathic generalized epilepsy. Seizure 1999;8:314–7.

264. Skardoutsou A, Voudris KA, Vagiakou EA. Non-convulsive status epilepticus associated with tiagabine therapy in children. Seizure 2003;12:599–601.

265. Ormrod D, McClellan K. Topiramate: a review of its use in childhood epilepsy. Paediatr Drugs 2001;3:293–319.

266. Lyseng-Williamson KA, Yang LP. Topiramate: a review of its use in the treatment of epilepsy. Drugs 2007;67:2231–56.

267. Reife R, Pledger G, Wu SC. Topiramate as add-on therapy: pooled analysis of randomized controlled trials in adults. Epilepsia 200;41 Suppl 1:S66–71.

268. Shank RP, Gardocki JF, Streeter AJ, Maryanoff BE. An overview of the preclinical aspects of topiramate: pharmacology, pharmacokinetics, and mechanism of action. Epilepsia 2000;41 Suppl 1:S3–9.

269. Perucca E. A pharmacological and clinical review on topiramate, a new antiepileptic drug. Pharmacol Res 1997;35:241–56.

270. Rosenfeld WE. Topiramate: a review of preclinical, pharmacokinetic, and clinical data. Clin Ther 1997;19:1294–308.

271. Coppola G, Capovilla G, Montagnini A, Romeo A, Spano M, Tortorella G, et al. Topiramate as add-on drug in severe myoclonic epilepsy in infancy: an Italian multicenter open trial. Epilepsy Res 2002;49:45–8.

272. Singh BK, White-Scott S. Role of topiramate in adults with intractable epilepsy, mental retardation, and developmental disabilities. Seizure 2002;11:47–50.

273. Wang Y, Zhou D, Wang B, Kirchner A, Hopp P, Kerling F, et al. Clinical effects of topiramate against secondarily generalized tonic-clonic seizures. Epilepsy Res 2002;49:121–30.

274. Dooley JM, Camfield PR, Smith E, Langevin P, Ronen G. Topiramate in intractable childhood onset epilepsy--a cautionary note. Can J Neurol Sci 1999;26:271–3.

275. Baeta E, Santana I, Castro G, Gon aS, Gon aT, Carmo I, et al. [Cognitive effects of therapy with topiramate in patients with refractory partial epilepsy.] Rev Neurol 2002;34:737–41.

276. Aldenkamp AP, Baker G, Mulder OG, Chadwick D, Cooper P, Doelman J, et al. A multicenter, randomized clinical study to evaluate the effect on cognitive function of topiramate compared with valproate as add-on therapy to carbamazepine in patients with partial-onset seizures. Epilepsia 2000;41:1167–78.

277. Zaccara G, Messori A, Cincotta M, Burchini G. Comparison of the efficacy and tolerability of new antiepileptic drugs: what can we learn from long-term studies? Acta Neurol Scand 2006;114:157–68.

278. Crawford P. An audit of topiramate use in a general neurology clinic. Seizure 1998;7:207–11.

279. Ojemann LM, Ojemann GA, Dodrill CB, Crawford CA, Holmes MD, Dudley DL. Language disturbances as side effects of topiramate and zonisamide therapy. Epilepsy Behav 2001;2:579–84.
280. Thompson PJ, Baxendale SA, Duncan JS, Sander JW. Effects of topiramate on cognitive function. J Neurol Neurosurg Psychiatry 2000;69:636–41.
281. Mula M, Trimble MR, Thompson P, Sander JW. Topiramate and word-finding difficulties in patients with epilepsy. Neurology 2003;60:1104–7.
282. Banta JT, Hoffman K, Budenz DL, Ceballos E, Greenfield DS. Presumed topiramate-induced bilateral acute angle-closure glaucoma. Am J Ophthalmol 2001;132:112–4.
283. Palmieri C, Canger R. Teratogenic potential of the newer antiepileptic drugs: what is known and how should this influence prescribing? CNS Drugs 2002;16:755–64.
284. Aldenkamp A, Vigevano F, Arzimanoglou A, Covanis A. Role of valproate across the ages. Treatment of epilepsy in children. Acta Neurol Scand Suppl 2006;184:1–13.
285. Johannessen CU, Johannessen SI. Valproate: past, present, and future. CNS Drug Rev 2003;9:199–216.
286. Loscher W. Valproate: a reappraisal of its pharmacodynamic properties and mechanisms of action. Prog Neurobiol 1999;58:31–59.
287. Hirsch E, Genton P. Antiepileptic drug-induced pharmacodynamic aggravation of seizures: does valproate have a lower potential? CNS Drugs 2003;17:633–40.
288. Harden CL, Meador KJ, Pennell PB et al. Practice parameter update: management issues for women with epilepsy--focus on pregnancy (an evidence-based review): teratogenesis and perinatal outcomes: report of the Quality Standards Subcommittee and Therapeutics and Technology Assessment Subcommittee of the American Academy of Neurology and American Epilepsy Society. Neurology 2009;73:133–41.
289. Tomson T, Battino D. Teratogenic effects of antiepileptic medications. Neurol Clin 2009;27:993–1002.
290. Chappell KA, Markowitz JS, Jackson CW. Is valproate pharmacotherapy associated with polycystic ovaries? Ann Pharmacother 1999;33:1211–6.
291. Isojarvi JI, Rattya J, Myllyla VV, Knip M, Koivunen R, Pakarinen AJ, et al. Valproate, lamotrigine, and insulin-mediated risks in women with epilepsy. Ann Neurol 1998;43:446–51.
292. Acharya S, Bussel JB. Hematologic toxicity of sodium valproate. J Pediatr Hematol Oncol 2000;22:62–5.
293. Genton P, Semah F, Trinka E. Valproic acid in epilepsy: pregnancy related issues. Drug Saf 2006;29:1–21.
294. Macdonald RL, Kelly KM. Antiepileptic drug mechanisms of action. Epilepsia 1995;36 Suppl 2:S2–12.
295. Coulter DA, Huguenard JR, Prince DA. Characterization of ethosuximide reduction of low-threshold calcium current in thalamic neurons. Ann Neurol 1989;25:582–93.
296. Yuen AW, Land G, Weatherley BC, Peck AW. Sodium valproate acutely inhibits lamotrigine metabolism. Br J Clin Pharmacol 1992;33:511–3.
297. Kramer G, Wohlrab G. Vigabatrin. In: Shorvon S, Perucca E, Engel JJr, eds. The treatment of epilepsy, 3nd edition, pp 699–712. Oxford: Wiley-Blackwell, 2009.
298. Willmore LJ, Abelson MB, Ben-Menachem E, Pellock JM, Shields WD. Vigabatrin: 2008 update. Epilepsia 2009;50:163–173.
299. Browne TR, Mattson RH, Penry JK, Smith DB, Treiman DM, Wilder BJ et al. Multicenter long-term safety and efficacy study of vigabatrin for refractory complex partial seizures: an update. Neurology 1991;41:363–364.
300. Arzimanoglou AA, Dumas C, Ghirardi L. Multicentre clinical evaluation of vigabatrin (Sabril) in mild to moderate partial epilepsies. French Neurologists Sabril Study Group. Seizure 1997;6:225–231.
301. Mumford JP, Dam M. Meta-analysis of European placebo controlled studies of vigabatrin in drug resistant epilepsy. Br J Clin Pharmacol 1989;27:101S–107S.
302. Beran RG, Berkovic SF, Buchanan N. A double-blind, placebo-controlled crossover study of vigabatrin 2 g/day and 3 g/day in uncontrolled partial seizures. Seizure 1996; 5: 259–265.
303. Connelly JF. Vigabatrin. Ann Pharmacother 1993;27:197–204.
304. French JA, Mosier M, Walker S, Sommerville K, Sussman N. A double-blind, placebo-controlled study of vigabatrin three g/day in patients with uncontrolled complex partial seizures. Vigabatrin Protocol 024 Investigative Cohort. Neurology 1996;46:54–61.
305. Eke T, Talbot JF, Lawden MC. Severe persistent visual field constriction associated with vigabatrin. BMJ 1997;314:180–1.
306. Chadwick D. Safety and efficacy of vigabatrin and carbamazepine in newly diagnosed epilepsy: a multicentre randomised doubleblind study. Vigabatrin European Monotherapy Study Group. Lancet 1999;354:13–9.
307. Lindberger M, Alenius M, Frisen L, Johannessen SI, Larsson S, Malmgren K, et al. Gabapentin versus vigabatrin as first add-on for patients with partial seizures that failed to respond to monotherapy: a randomized, double-blind, dose titration study. GREAT Study Investigators Group. Gabapentin in Refractory Epilepsy Add-on Treatment. Epilepsia 2000;41:1289–95.
308. French JA. Response: efficacy and tolerability of the new antiepileptic drugs. Epilepsia 2004;45:1649–51.
309. Glauser T, Ben-Menachem E, Bourgeois B, Cnaan A, Chadwick D, Guerreiro C, et al. ILAE treatment guidelines: evidence-based analysis of antiepileptic drug efficacy and effectiveness as initial monotherapy for epileptic seizures and syndromes. Epilepsia 2006;47:1094–120.

310. Panayiotopoulos CP, Agathonikou A, Sharoqi IA, Parker AP. Vigabatrin aggravates absences and absence status. Neurology 1997;49:1467.

311. Wild JM, Chiron C, Ahn H, Baulac M, Bursztyn J, Gandolfo E et al. Visual field loss in patients with refractory partial epilepsy treated with vigabatrin: final results from an open-label, observational, multicentre study. CNS Drugs 2009;23:965–982.

312. Gross-Tsur V, Banin E, Shahar E, Shalev RS, Lahat E. Visual impairment in children with epilepsy treated with vigabatrin. Ann Neurol 2000;48:60–4.

313. Duboc A, Hanoteau N, Simonutti M, Rudolf G, Nehlig A, Sahel JA, et al. Vigabatrin, the GABA-transaminase inhibitor, damages cone photoreceptors in rats. Ann Neurol 2004;55:695–705.

314. van der TK, Graniewski-Wijnands HS, Polak BC. Visual field and electrophysiological abnormalities due to vigabatrin. Doc Ophthalmol 2002;104:181–8.

315. Wroe SJ. Zonisamide. In: Shorvon S, Perucca E, Engel JJr, eds. The treatment of epilepsy, 3nd edition, pp 713–20. Oxford: Willey-Blackwell, 2009.

316. Willmore LJ, Seino M. International experiences and perspectives: zonisamide. Seizure 2004;13 Suppl 1:S1–72.

317. Chadwick DW, Marson AG. Zonisamide add-on for drug-resistant partial epilepsy. Cochrane Database Syst Rev 2002;(2):CD001416.

318. Baulac M. Introduction to zonisamide. Epilepsy Res 2006;68 Suppl 2:S3–9.

319. Tosches WA, Tisdell J. Long-term efficacy and safety of monotherapy and adjunctive therapy with zonisamide. Epilepsy Behav 2006;8:522–6.

320. Shinnar S, Pellock JM, Conry JA. Open-label, long-term safety study of zonisamide administered to children and adolescents with epilepsy. Eur J Paediatr Neurol 2009;13:3–9.

321. Arzimanoglou A, Rahbani A. Zonisamide for the treatment of epilepsy. Expert Rev Neurother 2006;6:1283–92.

322. Fukushima K, Seino M. A long-term follow-up of zonisamide monotherapy. Epilepsia 2006;47:1860–4.

323. Michael CT, Starr JL. Psychosis following initiation of zonisamide. Am J Psychiatry 2007;164:682.

324. Sills G, Brodie M. Pharmacokinetics and drug interactions with zonisamide. Epilepsia 2007;48:435–41.

Index

Page numbers followed by **b** indicate boxes.